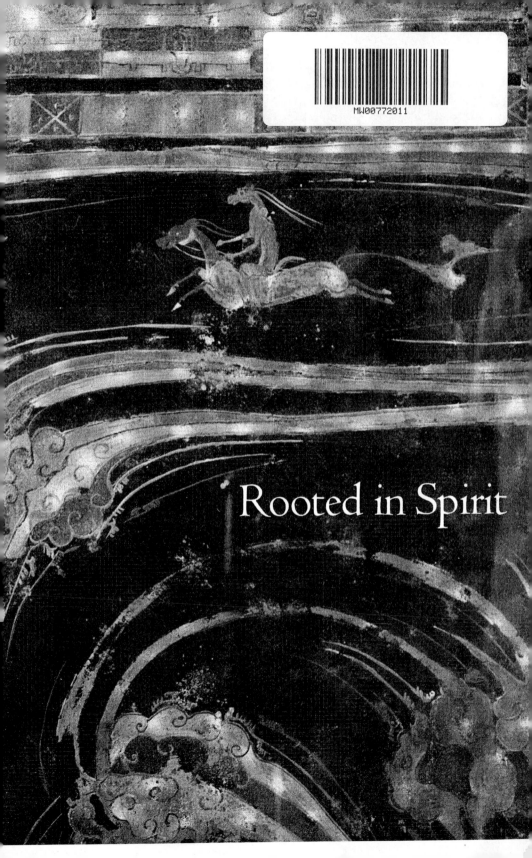

Rooted in Spirit

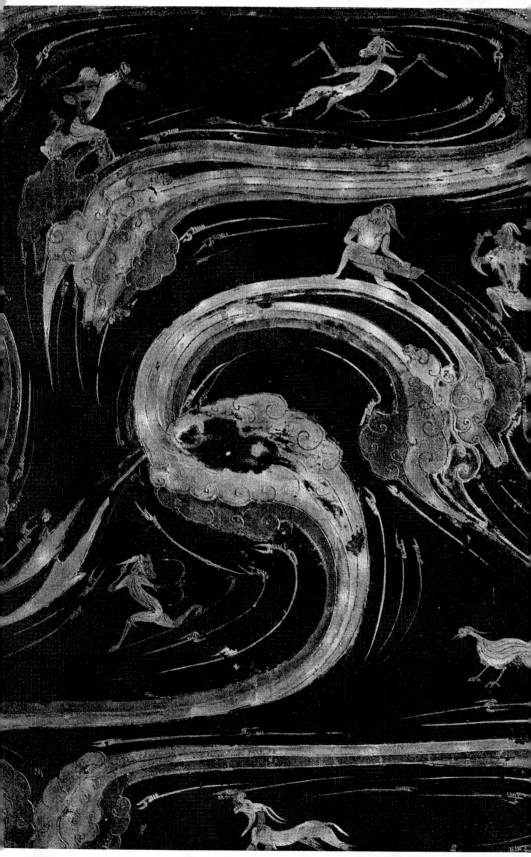

Rooted in Spirit

The Heart of Chinese Medicine

A sinological interpretation of
Chapter Eight of *Huangdi Neijing Lingshu*

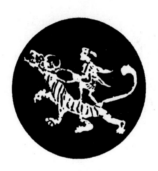

Translators from Chinese and Commentators
Claude Larre, S.J. & Elisabeth Rochat de la Vallée
Translator from French
Sarah Stang

Station Hill Press

Published by Station Hill Press, Inc., Barrytown, New York, 12507, in conjunction with the Institute for Publishing Arts, Inc., a not-for-profit, tax-exempt organization.

Cover and book design by Susan Quasha, assisted by Anastasia McGhee and Dominick Amarante.
Chinese characters by Yubo Wang.
Editorial development by George Quasha and Charles Stein.

Distributed by the Talman Company, 131 Spring Street, Suites 201E-N, New York, New York 10012

Library of Congress Cataloging-in Publication Data

Larre, Claude
    [*Mouvements du Coeur*. English]
Rooted in spirit : the heart of Chinese medicine / Claude Larre & Elisabeth Rochat de la Vallée ; translators for Chinese and commentators.
    p. cm.
    ISBN 0-88268-120-6 : $39.95. -- ISBN 0-88268-114-1 (pbk.) : $19.95
    1. Medicine, Chinese. 2. Mind and body. 3. Physician and patient. I. Rochat de la Vallée, Elisabeth. II. Title.
    R602.L37 1993
    615.5'3'0951--dc20   93-33271
                                                              CIP

Contents

Foreword

Rooted in Spirit is a translation of Chapter Eight of the *Lingshu* portion of the *Huangdi Neijing, The Yellow Emperor's Classic of Internal Medicine*, together with a commentary by contemporary French sinologists, Elisabeth Rochat de la Vallée and Claude Larre, S.J., and translated from the French by Sarah Stang.

Chapter Eight of the *Lingshu* gives an epitome of this metaphysical system and consequently shows the spiritual basis for the entire world of Chinese Medicine. In spite of this, the commonly held impression may be that Chinese medicine is fundamentally materialistic, though with a vitalistic bent; *Yin* and *Yang* may appear to be quasi-material principles, and one may easily overlook the elaborate and subtle relations between the bodily energies *(qi)* that animate the organ system, that rule the personality, the world of the Spirits *(shen)*, and the intercourse of Heaven and Earth, and provide the context for both the individual's state of health and the physician's intervention. As the practice of acupuncture, moxibustion, *qi gong*, and other Chinese healing arts that have their basis in the *Huangdi Neijing* become more familiar in the West, it is vitally important that the complete picture become more familiar as well, so that such a gross misunderstanding may be corrected. It is hoped that this translation and its commentary will serve these ends.

The Publisher

Translator's Note

The teaching that has provided the most fundamental grounding for my clinical practice of acupuncture, and to which I return again and again, is that of Claude Larre and Elisabeth Rochat de la Vallée. The notes and transcriptions from their semi-annual seminars in America and in England, and their translations of major chapters of the *Huangdi Neijing*, of *Zhuangzi* and of *Huainanzi* (and soon, hopefully, of *Laozi*), are the treasures in my library.

The words in the ancient Chinese texts are luminous guides for the living of my own life which becomes, in turn, the source from which I am able to serve and assist others. Members of the health care professions who are concerned with the interplay of the spirit with the emotions, mind, and body will find *Rooted in Spirit* (*Lingshu*, Chapter 8) a valuable resource providing models for creating and maintaining health, and also revealing pathology that can occur when the emotions and the spirit are not tended.

Père Larre and Madame Rochat de la Vallée continue the timeless tradition of adding commentaries to their translations, which are of especial value to Westerners in understanding the wisdom of the texts. These distinguished scholars of Chinese language and thought help us appreciate the power of the ancient Chinese approach to health by demonstrating the movement of life within the language itself, inseparable from the movement of life in living beings. They invite us to enlarge our understanding to the spiraling dimensions of Heaven and Earth and the Four Directions.

To place this document in its historical context, let me say that the the most famous of the ancient medical texts is the *Huangdi Neijing* (*Yellow Emperor's Classic of Internal Medicine*), a large part of which was written during the period of the Han Dynasty (206 B.C. - 220 A.D.) in the form of a dialogue between the Yellow Emperor and one or another of his ministers, of whom Qi Bo is the most famous. The Yellow Emperor asks questions about the nature of illness, and the answers offer models of harmony and balance for the maintenance of good health and the prevention of ill health. The *Neijing* has two parts: the *Suwen* (*Simple Questions*); and the *Lingshu* (*Spiritual Axis*), from which our present translation of Chapter 8 comes.

A note about the placement in the text of Chinese characters and their *pinyin* transliterations may be helpful. As a general rule the English word, the *pinyin*, and the character will be placed in that order, without commas or parentheses. The following example shows this presentation:

Blood and Breath *xue qi* 血氣, Essences and Spirits *jing shen* 精神 of man offer life and fulfill perfectly the natural destiny *xing ming* 性命 of each living being.

The *pinyin* Romanization of the Chinese characters is used throughout this translation, as *pinyin* is the current usage. For those readers who are more familiar with the Wade-Giles system of Romanization, Wade-Giles will be included in parentheses after the *pinyin* in the Glossary and in the two Indices, but not in the body of the text.

A comment should also be made concerning the English of this translation. The authors take words familiar to us and mount them contextually in such a way that the meaning is no longer so familiar. We are then forced to take another look beyond the comfortable limits of what we have understood up until now. Their usage of the words "Virtue," "Breath," "Knowing-how," "Intent," and "Will" are examples of this. These terms, as well as words like Essences, Spirits, Heart, Spleen, Liver, Kidneys, and Lung, will be capitalized in the beginning to indicate that in Chinese thought they have more extensive meanings than they do in ordinary English usage.[1] The words "Sage" and "Saint" will be used interchangeably throughout the text, when reference is made to a person who has attained the highest level of internal harmony.

Readers, you are challenged both to stretch and to surrender when entering the realm of *Lingshu* Chapter 8, and your commitment to do so will be richly rewarded.

Sarah Stang

---

[1] As the text progresses, however, the use of capital letters may be dispensed with in some instances, in order to avoid becoming too cumbersome.

Preface to the American Edition

It is untrue to say that the inscrutable Chinese are incapable of emotion. Why would there be such an abundance of minutely prescribed rituals for all family and social situations, if there were not an overflowing of something that needed to be contained? In Chinese theatre, novels, poetry, and even history, nothing occurs without tears, shouts, or sobs. Powerful feelings are expressed by torrential tears, by rages, by outbursts, and by brutal or secret revenges. Dishonor or shame disturbs hearts and makes them tremble. Chinese theatre resounds with curses, wounds, laughter, and love.

The Chinese have always been interested in observing the jolts of life which can be perceived in others, and which one also feels within oneself. They have researched the origin and the process of the movements that, exciting our feelings and transforming them into passions, direct our behaviors. They have isolated their effects and their capacity to devastate family and society, and also their power over an individual's life and over one's physical and mental health.

Rules or recipes for moderating the passions and making life calmer developed: asceticism, diet, gymnastics, rituals, etiquette, protocol, regulations of human and social relations. The accounts emphasized the effects of behavior, but always from the perspective of a man whose life unfolds between Heaven and Earth.

Heaven, which gives life, manifests the power and the Virtue that embrace all beings. Heaven penetrates Earth, whose breaths hasten to constitute corporeal forms, each according to its species. Heaven and Earth meet in the heart which is their designated place of *rendez-vous*. The essences coming from the mother and the father meet in an embrace that gives structure to the individual of the species; then the Spirits appear that guide the individual life.

As the Chinese saw it, the master-word of psychology is "heart." The heart is the vital center. It occupies the place of ruler. It is sacred vessel, holy land of each being; it welcomes the Spirits sent from Heaven. It contains and controls the Heaven/Earth exchange that makes us human and keeps us alive. By nature man's heart is vast and free like Heaven; always tempted to fill itself, it must seek to become empty.

Man's heart, involved naturally in knowledge coming from the senses and from the motion of the body, will from time to time close its shutters and withdraw. The art of the heart is mastery of life.

The *Lingshu* and the *Suwen* are two fundamental treatises of Chinese Medicine and have gained global seniority. *Lingshu* Chapter 8 exposes in several paragraphs what can be found in lengthy chapters of the other medical books and the general classical texts dealing with the operations of the heart. The Chapter 8 presentation is rigorous and systematic, placing the heart of man in the median position as both the end of the process of the constitution of a human being, and as the starting point of the correct expression and manifestation of the interior life of the being.

Its implacable descriptions show how the person held prey by passions unravels day after day, along the routes of deterioration implied by the particular passion that he has allowed to inhabit his heart.

We have translated the Chinese text as closely as possible. The commentary is broad; it tries to be simple and full of imagery. The American translation may occasionally give a strange tone to certain expressions or comparisons. We ask your pardon, dear reader, for the book you hold in your hand has already traveled through two worlds — from ancient China and present-day France — to come to you.

Introduction

Heaven gives and Earth receives. Heaven animates and Earth gives birth. Heaven sustains Earth with love and blesses her with light. The creative movement is called Virtue. The Virtue of Heaven falls upon Earth, penetrating and filling her. Sun and moon are witness to the heavenly Virtue.

> Heaven above, resplendent in your brilliance, you light the beams that come upon our earth.
>
> (*Book of Odes*, Part Two, *Xiaoya*, *Xiaoming* Ode)

Heaven invites, and Earth responds by receiving his Virtue. Earth's purpose is to form Breaths out of this Virtue from Heaven. Because of this community of Heaven/Earth life we can say: the Virtue of Earth is simply the transmitted Virtue of Heaven. We say the Breaths of Heaven because the Breaths produced must refer back to Heaven, to the origin of creative power. If we make a too-rigorous distinction between the Virtue of Heaven and the Breaths of Earth, we will ignore the work they accomplish together. However, it requires clarity, order, and care to articulate the value appropriate to each of the two operators of life. In Chapter 8 of the *Lingshu* we find, in a text of a few lines, seven propositions that articulate the bringing about of the penetration of man's heart by the Virtue of Heaven.

Huangdi, the Yellow Emperor, man of the past, is the man of forever. Having stepped across the boundaries of his earthly life (when "initiated and perfect, he rose to the sky" [cf. *Suwen*, Chapter 1, in *The Way of Heaven*]), he pursues his role as teacher of all that lives under Heaven; he remains the solicitous Prince caring for all his people, and he is the model for the living. The life of the Yellow Emperor Huangdi is our own life as it is when we realize our destiny. Our nature, paths, and goals are individualized, but the final destination is Heaven (already attained by our ancestors), to which we are summoned by our heart.

The origin of the inexhaustible Source, an "imperceptible thread indefinitely spun" (*Laozi*, Chapter 6), is the miraculous effectiveness of the Spirits. The place to look for the source of the living is in "the birth of Heaven and Earth." The Spirits come from Heaven and consent to remain within a man only if his heart is as serene and empty as Heaven itself.

Huangdi's great vitality as an infant, seen through the expression of his Breaths, was due only to the presence of the Spirits. All that was "marvelous" in his expression was conferred upon him by the Spirits. As he grew in age, going from nursling to child, he was noticed for the fairness of his conduct. This quality must be attributed to the Spirits that always firmly maintain the direction of life despite the internal tensions of adolescence. In its turn, adolescence bears its own fruit (the adult), and the Spirits are still in command of the personality: they guarantee what we call moral qualities. Chapter 1 of the *Suwen* speaks of "loyalty and sagacity," qualities required of a King of the universe.

The human terrestrial adventure is over when, through initiation and the asceticism that leads to perfection, the man ready for the heavenly ride is released by the high movement of the Spirits and withdrawn from visible, earthly involvement.

The Atmosphere of Rooted in Spirit

We attempt here to render an interpretation that reveals as nearly as possible the breadth of the Chinese reflection which trembles with admiration for the workings of life, constant with a constancy whose cost is constant change.

A painter often animates the solitude of high mountain forests, suggesting a violent and brilliant waterfall hurtling and plunging there. Painters also like to depict the Yi Chang rapids on the Great River. We know that the most richly silted waters come from Heaven.

> Friend, don't you see that the waters of the Yellow River
> Come down from Heaven and hasten toward the sea?
> *Li Bo*

Water is the manifestation of Heaven. This power also falls within us, "in an equally silent thunder." We call it "Virtue." This Virtue brings to life, develops, and maintains the movement of each being. Its gift and receipt can be an observable, visible phenomenon. In its invisible aspect, it is the mystery to be contemplated, as if we were standing before a latticed doorway. (In order to see [through it], we must know how to position ourselves, and how to receive the image that comes to our eyes.) The expanding power that stops right here, to make me into a being, can be compared to the cascading of the waters from Heaven.[2]

---

[2] *Cascade* is the title of the French edition of *Rooted in Spirit*. In order to preserve the rich imagery of the power of Heaven pouring down upon all beings like a waterfall, the two sections of this book will be entitled Cascade I and Cascade II.

Here and there this gushing can be seen. The continuity of the impetus (of the *yang* movement) can be perceived in the changes, appearing as transformations. We think of a rocky basin where the fallen splashing water collects and then escapes through a channel. The twisting of its particular course may push the water on in torrents, or stop it in ponds. The earth may drink and absorb the water, or move it on in clever irrigation of gardens and fields, until it joins the sea and the air before its return to Heaven. Throughout all these transformations, water remains the Virtue that gives life. (This calls to mind the *klepsudra*, or water-clock. The full upper bowl overflows to activate the lower one. From level to level, the water descends the steps, marking out the time. Whereas time thus ensues mechanically, its duration is born from changes and transformations.) The proud Virtue of Heaven consents to become the humble virtue of a man. There are thirteen stages, thirteen ideograms, to indicate the changes and transformations. Where they meet — the theatre of exchange, the *rendez-vous* of the Spirits that hasten forth from Heaven — is the place where my life is rooted. This place is "I" *wo* 我, "my heart" *wo xin* 我心.

The Title: Ben Shen (*Rooting in the Spirits*)

In aspiring to the heights of ancient thought which was always concerned with Heaven and Man, we must not abandon the approaches to the Way "so smooth, so wide, to which people prefer the tortuous paths" (cf. *Laozi*, Chapter 53). In order not to miss the scope of the teaching, we must return to its essence: to ease and heal, all that one can do is delicately return to the celestial current (by means of the therapy used) that which lives only by the ceaseless going and coming of the Spirits. The editor of the *Lingshu* evidently gave the title *Ben Shen* to Chapter 8 in order to take the movement of the breaths within us and place it definitively under the authority of the Spirits, and in order to raise to the level of "knowing-how",[3] all those informed by spiritual quality.[4]

---

[3] The knowledge of how to manage things, and especially of how to manage one's own life (see characters 84-186, line 30 and following commentary).

[4] Chapters 2 (*Ben Shu*) and 8 (*Ben Shen*) of the *Lingshu* share a common aspect in summoning the practitioner to the roots of life in order to understand how life works and how, from the meeting of two essences, life organizes and differentiates itself. Chapter 2 explains how and where the resources of animation proper to an

An 8th Chapter: the 13th-14th century rescension of the *Lingshu* upon which this text is based, gives the 8th place to the *Ben Shen* chapter. But in other compilations of medical texts, classified presentations of the *Lingshu* and the *Suwen*, it is assigned to more commanding positions:

—In the *Zhenjiu jiayijing* (which appeared in 259 A.D.) it begins the work. When people become aware of its contents, they will see that it was logical to use *Lingshu* Chapter 8 to introduce the themes representing the essential points of the *Neijing*.

—In the *Huangdi neijing taisu*, by Yang Shangshan (6th-7th century A.D.), it appears at the head of the section consecrated to the *zang/fu* (viscera/organs).

General Organization of the Text

Chapter 8 of the *Lingshu* contains 644 characters. Its title, *Ben Shen*, reminds us that pricking with a needle is effective only when accomplished by the hand of an acupuncturist whose Spirit can go all the way to the heart of animation, to the Spirits of the patient. Qi Bo, the heavenly Master, answers Huangdi methodically and at length. In Huangdi's question two lines of interrogation intersect. One is similar to that in Chapter 1 of the *Suwen*: "When man, who is produced by the Virtue of Heaven, becomes unsettled, is it the fault of man or of Heaven?" The other interrogation is a methodical review of the vocabulary used to set forth, according to their successive generation, the thirteen instances of the inner life that specifically attest that the Virtue of Heaven in the Heart of man has become a Knowing-how. It is a Knowing-how nourished by Reflection and supported by the power and the clarity of Will and Intent. Such mastery of life is required in order for the Spirit as well as the hand of the acupuncturist to know how to find the Spirits (of the patient). But it seems that the presentation of developments in the way a man's Spirits can be wounded by attacks from the passions — even to death itself — may be also a methodic review of the general teaching. Sensitive to this organization of the text around

---

individual lie in the body. This chapter also gives more specific details as to how and where the connections are arranged for the interplay between the most internal agents of life and the most external ones. Chapter 8 explains the way numerous functions join in a single life under the guidance and powerful drive of the Spirits.

two systematizations (that of the thirteen instances ruled by the heart, and that of the relationship of the emotions, the seasons, and the *zang*), we have divided our presentation into two parts:

Cascade I   (CHARACTERS 1-226)
Cascade II   (CHARACTERS 227-644)

Outline of the Text
Cascade I
(CHARACTERS 1–226)

The Way of Heaven, through the Virtue of Heaven and the Breaths of Earth, institutes Knowing-how in every person, by means of thirteen steps. The Heart takes charge of the Beings.[5] One can attain long life and everlasting vision through the Heart.

char. 1-83: Huangdi's opening statement followed by the double question addressed to Qi Bo:
  A. Who is responsible for the disorder in the vital proceedings?
  B. How does the Heavenly Virtue become, in me, an effectual practical knowing?

char. 84-226: Qi Bo's answer, given in two parts (char. 87-186 for part A, and char. 187-226 for part B):
  A. The thirteen instances of the inner life:
      1. Virtue of Heaven
      2. Breaths of Earth
      3. Emergence of Living Beings
      4. Arrival of the Essences
      5. Appearance of the Spirits
      6. Movements of the *Hun*
      7. Subservient movements of the *Po*
      8. The Heart receives the Virtue of Heaven;
         The Heart watches over the Spirits, just as the Spirits guard the Heart
      9. Intent
     10. Will
     11. Thought

---

[5] The Ten Thousand Beings, everything under Heaven.

Cascade II
(CHARACTERS 227–644)

The attack on the Spirits releases the passions. The Five *Zang* are affected, and the perturbed processes of life lead the organism to premature death, which intervenes at the season in question. There is an examination of the emptiness and fullness of Breaths in the Five *Zang* and a description of the correlative symptoms.

char. 227–292: Specific aspects of the pathology of the Spirits.

char. 293–444: The way each of the Five *Zang* is affected by the pathology of the Spirits (*Shen*, Intent, *Hun*, *Po*, Will), and the reaction of the body to each situation.

char. 445–463: How the Essences are attacked and how the body reacts.

char. 464–492: The *zang* must be preserved from attack in order to avoid death through the absence of Breaths.

char. 493–527: In a pathological situation one must needle only if there are signs of the presence of Essences and Spirits, and if there is a favorable outlook.

char. 528–644: In taking care of someone, one must know how to recognize the pathological emptiness or fullness particular to each of the Five *Zang*, and the manifestations of the correlative disorders.

Cascade I

Huangdi puts this question to Qi Bo:

For every needling, the method is above all
Not to miss the rooting in the Spirits.

Xue and *Mai*, *Ying* and *Qi*, *Jing* and *Shen*,
These are stored by the Five *Zang*.   5

If a situation becomes such that
By a succession of overflowings and total invasion
They leave the *Zang*,
Then the Essences are lost;
And *Hun* and *Po* are carried away in an
uncontrollable agitation,   10
Will and Intent become confused and disordered.
Knowing-how and Reflection abandon us.

Where does this state come from?
Should Heaven be blamed? Is it Man's fault?

And what do we call Virtue, Breaths, Life, Essences,
  Shen, *Hun*, *Po*,   15
Heart, Intent, Will, Thought, Knowing-How, Reflection?

Characters 1 to 83

黃帝問於歧伯曰
huang di wen yu qi bo yue

凡刺之法先必本於神
fan ci zhi fa xian bi ben yu shen

血脈營氣精神
xue mai ying qi jing shen

此五臟之所藏也
ci wu zang zhi suo cang ye

至其淫泆離臟則精失
zhi qi yin yi li zang ze jing shi

魂魄飛揚
hun po fei yang

志意恍亂
zhi yi huang luan

智慮去身者
zhi lü qu shen zhe

何因而然乎
he yin er ran hu

天之罪與人之過乎
tian zhi zui yu ren zhi guo hu

何謂德氣生精神魂魄心意志思智慮
he wei de qi sheng jing shen hun po xin yi zhi si zhi lü

請問其故
qing wen qi gu

For every needling, the method is above all
Not to miss the rooting in the Spirits. (lines 2-3)

Human activity, from beginning to end (the end being simply our return to the origin), is directed by the Spirits. The quality of life and the fullness of our years are assured only by association with them. We must therefore remember that the root of life is in the Spirits. Root is *ben* 本, and the Spirits are *shen* 神.

What do the Spirits, the *shen*, do? They lead *yu* 御 the Breaths *qi* 氣. The Breaths within me are not undifferentiated; they are individualized. The aspect of individualization is called the Essences *jing* 精.

In Chapter 1 of the *Suwen*, Chapters 1 and 24 of *Zhuangzi*, Chapter 1 of *Huainanzi*, and doubtless in many other texts, life is spoken of as a rambling walk directed by the Spirits. Throughout the body the Breaths are guided appropriately if we allow the Spirits to lead the parade and take us with them.

The association of Spirits with Breaths *shen qi* 神氣 is reflected in a living being and becomes perceptible as emptiness or fullness. We speak of fullness or emptiness of the *zang* (viscera) and/or the *fu* (organs/bowels), as a rise in power and/or decline of Breaths and Blood. Before inserting a needle, one observes the situation and reads the visible signs for a tendency towards an absence or progressive loss of the Essences/Spirits *jing shen* 精神. One then conducts one's treatment according to the result of this observation.

Huangdi is the Emperor of all the living. He embraces the breadth of possible interventions that organize themselves around the amazingly effective Pivot: the needle and the *Lingshu*. He reminds us: "Above all do not miss the rooting in the Spirits." Indeed, the concrete reality of life, the object of both glance and needle, is the Breaths animated by the Spirits. Blood appears as an abode of the Spirits, and the Essences as a specification for the Breaths. All is taken into account in the needling, whose effect goes straight to the Spirits, our true masters.

We speak of conduct of life. We could be more precise and say that the Spirits, sent abundantly and permanently to me by Heaven, hold the reins of the Breaths that constitute me. These Spirits are pleased to stay when they feel welcomed. They function conjointly with the Essences. It is natural to them to follow the seasons and to cause beings to behave in ways that help the harmony of the correct Breaths to be maintained. Health can always hit a snag from an irregularity that the environment can bring on, that a person's encumbered heart can provoke, and that the bad times one is living in can multiply. If the harmony is not re-established by itself, the needle may intervene in a situation that threatens to become critical, to avoid permanent installation of perverse Breaths. To be effective, and at the same time not violate the organism, the acupuncturist goes all the way to the origin of the patient's life, to that place where the Spirits are rooted, to *ben shen* 本神.

Xue and Mai, Ying and Qi, Jing and Shen, (line 4)

The Six Authorities that make up the life of a Being can be grouped in three pairs: (1) *xue mai*, (2) *ying qi*, and (3) *jing shen*.

(1) *Xue Mai*. Blood *xue* 血 and the pathways of animation *mai* 脉,[6] constitute the network holding the circulation that maintains life in the body under the direction of the Spirits. It is the power of *jue yin*, because the Liver (*jue yin* of the foot) stores the blood, and because the Heart has mastery *xin zhu* 心主, (*jue yin* of the hand) over the pathways of animation. The *jue yin* aspect of life is in the circulation of an exact amount of blood, rich in essences, but also in the Spirits whose benefits are spread everywhere by the network. It is the beginning of what becomes the *yang* aspect of life in its gushing forth and spreading out. (Liver and Heart are the two *yang*, or masculine, *zang*, corresponding to Wood and Fire.)

(2) *Ying Qi*. This is the organization, completion, construction, and reconstruction of the vitality of the being, especially through nutrition *ying* 營, and integration of the Breaths *qi* 氣. These Breaths provide, *par excellence*, the *yang* aspect of defense, and also take part in the maintenance of life. It is the power of the *tai yin* through the Spleen (*tai yin* of the foot) which is the center of nutritive distributions, transforming and assimilating and reconstituting to the farthest extremity, and through the Lung (*tai yin* of the hand) which has mastery of the Breaths, and whose power radiates all the way to the body's boundaries (the skin and the body hair). The *tai yin* aspect is the maintenance of vitality within an exact harmony that guards within the interior all that rebuilds, and sends out to the exterior all that solidifies the defense (the

---

[6] *Mai*, pathways and network of (and for) animation. The *mai* are also the pulses. In some literature *mai* is translated as meridians.

strength of the guards). It is the only guarantee of correct *yang* diffusion toward the exterior.

(3) *Jing Shen* are the mystery of life. The Spirits *shen* 神 impregnate the essences *jing* 精; they create life and give it duration.

It is the strength of the *shao yin*, because the Kidneys (*shao yin* of the foot) are the base where the essences are composed and re-composed, and because the Heart (*shao yin* of the hand) by its emptiness, can be the dwelling-place of the Spirits. It is the high and deep relationship of Heaven (Heart) and Earth (Kidneys) that operates this living mystery. Heaven/Earth in movement is seen in that which descends from on high in the image of good, of Virtue, of solar fire (Heaven), and in that which ascends from below in the image of water rising, of clouds (Earth). This is the relation of the Essences to the Spirits. Life exists only through their joining and their co-penetration. Animation without form is as impossible as form without animation.

The authors of the *Lingshu* visualize nothing less than the Great Acupuncturist. They know that the good practitioner's diagnosis is a connection from deep within himself to the Spirits of the patient, which are showing signs recognizable to the practitioner. There is free com-munication between Spirits. The signs perceived by the acupuncturist are the different observable states of the Breaths, which themselves depend on the Essences. The attentive and properly oriented human spirit quickly and infallibly interprets the rapport of the Essences/ Spirits *jing shen*. Thus he goes at once to the seat of the malady, which will be the place where he intervenes. As an artisan modulates the pressure of his engraving tool on the ivory, the acupuncturist pru-dently, but without the least hesitation, controls the manner and the power of his gesture. This is what permits him to go with his Spirits to the Spirits of the patient. This is what makes his work a master-piece: the faultless fulfillment of infallible inspiration.

Each time that this deep level where the Essences/Spirits reside is touched by the healer, the vitality *ying qi* is restored. In this coupled expression, *ying* represents the aspect of organization of the Breaths and the advancement of the vital movement, and *qi* calls forth the Breaths and, more particularly, the aspect of life that defends itself from all perverse attacks. A clear distinction is made in the classical text: there is a quality of Essences/Spirits, and there is a quality of

ying/qi. It is a way of saying that the individual in question is in ___
health. In the tradition, things appear with a redundancy that can
nevertheless be an interesting re-statement. Certainly, without a good
rapport between *ying* and *qi*, the combative forces of life are neither
powerful enough nor well-enough defended. The ultimate reason for
the existence of such a state (poor *ying/qi* rapport) is that the liaison
between the Essences and Spirits is deficient. The acupuncturist's
gesture should be directed there. If he himself lacks *jing shen* and is
without a high level of Essences/Spirits, he will not search deeply
enough in his patient for the disease — all the way to the rooting of
the *ying/qi* vitality, to the Spirits.

Without exaggerating, one might have the feeling that the acupuncturist adapts himself, with his needles, to the conditions in which he
finds the *ying/qi* of the patient. He knows he can intervene — with an
effect that can be immediate or slow — in the present state of the
vitality, with the certainty that the Essence/Spirit relationship will
touch the vitality with the seal of spirituality. In the etymological sense
of the term, health is thus strengthened.

The vitality is seen and felt in the quality of animation of the
Breaths, and in the turnover in the circulation of the Blood. That is the
main interest of the first consideration of *xue/mai*. One must see and
palpate before needling. Then one knows where and how to proceed.

Inspection by a practised eye, palpation, and especially the taking
of the pulses *mai* 脉, reveal the state of the patient. The eye and fingers
receive a sensitive projection of the network of Blood which is the
dwelling-place of the Spirits.

The Great Acupuncturist, manipulating the needle, goes all the way
to the Spirits. The progression in three stages exposes a process, but
the acupuncturist treats according to both his immediate grasp of the
patient, and the visualization of his own Spirits.

Chapter 8 of the *Lingshu* shows a series of six terms: Blood *xue* and
the Pathways of Animation *mai*; Maintenance *ying* and the Breaths *qi*;
the Essences *jing* and the Spirits *shen*. These constitute the totality of
the treasure stored by the Five *Zang*.

Another series of the six terms are given in the *Neijing*, in regard
to the storing function of the Five *Zang*, as follows:

> The Five *Zang* are for the storage of Essences/Spirits *jing
> shen* 精神, Blood and Breaths *xue qi* 血氣, the *Hun* 魂 and
> *Po* 魄
>
> *Lingshu*, Chapter 47

In a different context, here is still another series of six terms: Essences *jing*; Breaths *qi*; bodily liquids and fluids *jin* 津 ; more dense bodily liquids *ye* 液 ; Blood *xue*; and Pathways of Animation *mai*. In this way Chapter 30 of *Lingshu* clarifies a single Breath, under another pattern of six denominations.

These are stored by the Five Zang. (line 5)

The movement from Five to Six is demonstrated here.

Life both makes itself and regenerates itself through storing; it spends and deploys from its storehouse. An interiority is expressed. The Chinese system of numerology gives evidence of endogenous and exogenous transformations. Uneven (Heavenly) numbers mark the successive aspects of interiorness from the simplest to the most complex, and represent to our spirits that which is truly produced in the universe. The even (terrestrial) numbers are the unfolding of the uneven numbers. Through them the unions, extensions, relations, gyrations, influences and totalities of correspondences are made. But the powerful mystery of That Which Exists is always present there, in the bosom of all the vital transformations. There is no less unity in the Chinese pair than in the Chinese singular, no less unity contained in the Four Sides of the Earth, in the Four Seas that join them, and in The Four Seasons that accumulate their breaths, than there is in the harmonized breath resulting from the interpenetration of *yin/yang* (and from all the homologous interpenetrations governing the universal reference to everything that is under the mastery of Three). For a complete analysis one might refer to Marcel Granet, whose writings on the subject have not been surpassed.

For our purposes here, it suffices to recall that the number Five is the number of thesaurization, or storing *cang* 藏 . Five instances, called the Five *Zang* 臓 , accumulate (each according to its specific nature) the Essences that are the framework of life of the human species. Now with respect to the different re-groupings in the six terms mentioned above (since the text says that these are "stored by the Five *Zang*"), we are tempted to succumb to games of correspondence. It is difficult to keep from trying to give to each *zang* an affinity with one of the grouped instances in the scheme of Six. Rightly so. The same principle applies to the most important of the correlations: fixing the relationship of the Five *Zang* and the Six *Fu*. The difficulty is simply in reconciling, without artifice and without forcing things, the lightly divergent presentations of the rapport between the Five *Zang* and the Six Authorities (*xue, mai, ying, qi, jing, shen*). We refer the reader to Chapters 23 and 62 of the *Suwen*. However, the surest and most complete reference is at the end of Chapter 8 of the *Lingshu*:

> The Liver stores the Blood *xue*. . . . The Spleen stores the principle of Maintenance *ying*. . . . The Heart stores the Network of Animation *mai*. . . . The Lung stores the Breaths *qi*. . . . The Kidneys store the Essences *jing*. . . .

Here we find five of the six terms of the ensemble that we are studying. The term that is missing is the Spirits (*shen*). There is a reason for this absence. When the Heart stores the *mai* it is a question of the Heart's exercising its mastery; but the same Heart is the dwelling-place of the Spirits, an empty space for the return to unity of all the differentiated aspects of life.

"Overflowings" and *"Invasions"* (cf lines 6-9)

Overflowings and invasions are expressed in Chinese as *yin yi* 淫泆.

Yin 淫 (in this instance) is debauchery, turning away from the good path. Appropriate and correct conduct becomes licentious and twisted. There is an infiltration that distorts whatever it penetrates. The "Six Infiltrations" *liu yin* 六淫 are the way in which the six atmospheric Breaths (cold, heat, humidity, dryness, wind, fire) become perverted and penetrate the poorly defended human body, to debauch and divert the correct Breaths of the organism.

Yi 泆 is an overflowing. The river no longer flows tranquilly in its bed, but the torrential waters ravage everything, cover everything. Passions no longer have dikes, nor does capriciousness have limits; life is dissolute.

Here the coupling *yin yi* marks the rupture of dikes and dams at the level of conduct, feelings, passions, and desires. One gives oneself up to all excesses because one is no longer held in the straight line of life. Life and its movements no longer follow the natural course but burst out in a disastrous way.

The expression *yin yi* is ancient. The *Yueji* ("Memoir of Music," part of the *Liji, Book of Rites*) shows how daily hazards can disorganize life. A prince loses mastery of himself, rebellions burst out, disorders lead to the collapse of the dynasty and the ruin of the empire. The Heart, no longer ruling anything, brings about the loss — indeed, the death — of the individual. Things pass easily from the level of the feelings to the level of the breaths, when the external perverse breaths introduce themselves silently into the correct breaths to "turn them around," to pervert them.

> It is a fact that the (Ten Thousand) Beings provoke in a person an indefinite series of reactions *gan* 感 . The incapacity to master the attractions and repulsions that are born in contact with a Being produce the transformations and alterations *hua* 化 that the beings *wu* 物 bring about in a person.
>
> A person transformed by beings loses his celestial disposition *tian li* 天理, and he is filled with human lusts *yu* 欲 . The rebellious Heart, false and deceitful, revolts; the disturbed conduct becomes dissolute *yin yi* 淫泆 and generates disorders *zuo luan* 作亂.
>
> *Yueli*

In losing one's own command center, one is completely lost. By the light poured into it by the Spirits, this center alone could lead our life along the line of its natural harmonious development. This center alone is responsible for our good health.

To lose one's own being is to lose the internal storage of the essences that give themselves to the Spirits. This loss allows exterior incitements to cause the disappearance of what should remain deeply stored for building and re-building the being.

One who lets himself be thus circumvented will not be able to reclaim himself after a certain time, because the very foundations of the powers that could have allowed a reprise have been permitted to escape.

The Serenity of a Sage

The Sage is not touched by external seductions; his joy of life is anchored in his self-possession, which is the only thing worth possessing in the world. It is the opposite of dispossession of self, which comes from the illusion of possessing something. Who would speak of possessing furtive pleasures? This idea is illustrated in Chapter 1 of *Huainanzi*:

The expression "find oneself" *zi de* 自得 [7] means conserv-

---

[7] To possess oneself.

ing the integrity of the personal being *quan qi shen* 全其身
Union with the Dao is the way to find/possess oneself.

Let us imagine a pleasure cruise along the banks of a great river
or the seashore, or riding the great steed Niao, shaded by a
canopy decorated with martin-fisher feathers, watching the
military dance of the plumed helmets, to the strains of Wuxiang
music. Our ears are charmed by the tunes of Daolang, Qilu,
Jizhen, or performances of tunes from Cheng and Wei, or
popular warblings of the light music from Chu.

Imagine hunting high-flying birds in the many marshy
tributaries of the great river, or hunting big game in the
Yuanyou park.

These are pleasures that excite the populace and open the
floodgates to all loose living *yin yi.*

If a Sage finds himself involved, there is nothing there that can
divert his vital spirit *jing shen,* [8] put his free choice *qi zhi* 氣誌[9]
into disarray, disturb his Heart, attack his psyche *qing
xing* 情性.[10]

The upsetting of life's conditions, blows received, and violence experienced must not trouble the regularity of life's internal movements for
very long:

The Sage would adopt (any life imposed upon him) without sadness or recrimination, and without losing his good
humor and contentment *zi le* 自樂 .[11] Why? Because his
intimate being *nei* 内 possesses the means to communicate
with the machinery (organization) of the world *tong yu tian
ji* 通於天機 in such a way that wealth, honor, leisure — or
their opposites — are incapable of affecting the power of his
soul *zi de* 自得 .[12] In the same way the cawing of the crow
or the cooing of the turtle-dove does not change with cold or
scorching heat, dryness or humidity.

He who possesses the Dao has become master of himself

---

[8] Essences/Spirits.
[9] His Breaths and his will.
[10] His feelings and his own nature.
[11] The joy that is naturally within.
[12] Possession of oneself.

and holds himself beyond the influence of things that are in perpetual motion, for it is neither timing nor luck that gives him his self-possession *zi de*. By 'self-possession' we mean that the individual soul living at the interior of a specific nature *xing ming zhi qing* 性命之情 holds himself in that which constitutes his repose *an* 安 . . . .

Huainanzi, Chapter 1

Through contrary conduct one is lost; he lets go of his Essences; something is missing, and at all levels of vitality there is disorder.

The *Hun* and the *Po* are expressions of the Spirits. When this disorder exists, the *Hun* fly away like birds that nothing can hold; the *Po* stir about thoughtlessly in the absence of effective control and the actual presence of the Spirits.

Will and Intent lose the intimate and harmonious relationship that allows them to be the basis for constructing the mental world. They no longer control the situation as they should, as mediators and adjuncts of the Heart. Instead, they let disorder triumph.

Knowing-how and Reflection are the natural ways of a sound internal vitality which is well-constructed, well-directed, and well-heeded. If the source of life runs dry in the interior, how can it still produce the effects of Knowing-how and Reflection? No longer does anything exact or pertinent come from this being.

The *Neijing* deals ceaselessly with the subject of the being as the prey of perdition. Being a medical treatise and not specifically a treatise of moral philosophy, it shows how these outbursts injure health, and it describes them in very physical terms.

The Demented are Lost *(cf lines 10-12)*

When obsessive thoughts *si xiang* 思想 hold sway indefinitely and one does not obtain what one aspires to, when the Intent *yi* 意 flows out uncontrolled *yin* 淫 to the exterior and one spends one's intensity in the bedroom, the ancestral muscle *zong jin* 宗筋 becomes completely spent. This causes muscular impotence *jin wei* 筋痿 to the point where there is uncontrollable leaking of the white substance *bai yin* 白淫.

Suwen, Chapter 44

A breakdown in the conduct of the life of the Spirits brings perversion into the thinking process, which repeats itself, becomes obstinate, digs in — and the "Intent" is stricken, is led astray, and is no longer controlled by the internal Spirits of the Heart. Consequently, this estrangement shows up in life's activities. In the shock of rebound, what holds the power of life internally also fails. There is no retention; one has lost control of oneself, and from this there is leakage which can become spermatorrhea and white discharge.

Hun and *po*, Will and Intent, maintenance and defense, and Essences/Spirits are the four couplings whose balance composes life. The strength in unity that makes it possible for the members of each of these couples to cooperate with each other comes from the omnipresence of the Spirits, kept in the Heart and represented everywhere by messengers *shi* 使 who are envoys from the Heart. This is the rooting in the Spirits.

A text from Chapter 14 of the *Suwen* clarifies this notion:

> Huangdi: "What is the breakdown of the body and the complete anemia that leads to the incapacity to do anything worthwhile?"
>
> Qi Bo answered: "The Spirits *shen* no longer function *shi* 使.
>
> The Emperor continued: "What does 'the Spirits no longer function' mean?"
>
> Qi Bo replied: "Metal or stone needles are on the level of the Way *dao* 道. When the Essences/Spirits *jing shen* cannot enter, when the Will and Intent *zhi yi* 志意 cannot be maintained appropriately, then the disease cannot be cured. For when the Essences are deteriorated and the Spirits have gone away *qu* 去, neither the deep maintenance *ying* 營 nor the defense *wei* 衛 can return and be recovered. How does that happen? When desires and lusts are renewed indefinitely, along with a pusillanimous fear that cannot be stopped, the Essences/Breaths *jing qi* 精氣 loosen their hold until there is ruination. The *ying* 營 congeals and the *wei* 衛 is torn away. Then the Spirits leave us and the illness is incurable."

Knowing-how and reflection are the other end of the chain: the good conduct of life, acts and behavior, the interdependence of actions and reactions. They are like nourishment and protection (*ying wei)*, on a psychological level.

Will and intent serve as intermediary between the two. This is not the highest level, but as it relates to particular features unique to a man's life, these are the authorities that command and regulate. The beginning of Chapter 3 of the *Suwen* points this out:

> When the Breaths of Azure Heaven are clear and serene,
> will and intent *zhi yi* govern *zhi* 治 (themselves) (appropri-
> ately). As a result of following this good lead, the *yang* breaths
> are solid, and even robbers and perversities can do no harm.

Correctness in the governing of a being comes from the cooperation and stability of will and intent. In addition, in this coupling of will and intent, we find a relationship between the Kidneys and Spleen, be-tween the representative authorities of Anterior Heaven, and those representing Posterior Heaven. The remainder of Chapter 8 of the *Lingshu* returns to this question.

Where Lies the Blame? (cf lines 13-14)

The question – whether this condition is caused by the man who has allowed it to settle in him, or whether it is a phenomenon of human nature – is not purely rhetorical.

Man has a heart, feelings, and passions. Such a nature could inher-ently allow itself to be carried away by human passions, unable to do anything to stop it. Some might resist it and others not, no matter what; it would depend on the individual nature of each. All are not given the same strength of character, the same spiritual quality, the same resis-tance to the passions, or the same fierceness in attaining their desires. Can a man really be considered guilty, or even ill, because his passions and desires direct his life?

This question will not be answered. Rather, Qi Bo, with conciseness and authority, will satisfy Huangdi by giving a terse definition for each of the thirteen aspects he has been asked to explain. These definitions allow us to see rapidly, faultlessly, and without haste, the composition of life and its development. Life is known by its roots in the world of Spirits, and by what is nearest to the Spirits – the emergence of man: the spiritual, psychic, intellectual, mental, and emotional world. Through these thoughts an answer to the first part of Huangdi's question will be suggested indirectly: how can degradation leading to collapse be explained; and how can man's clear responsibility to call on the Spirits be visualized?

Qi Bo Replied:

Heaven within me is Virtue.
Earth within me is the Breaths.
Virtue flows down, the Breaths expand,
    and there is life.   20
The coming forth of living beings indicates the Essences.
The embrace of the two Essences indicates the Spirits.
That which follows the Spirits faithfully in their going
    and coming indicates the *Hun*.
That which associates with the Essences in their exiting
    and entering indicates the *Po*.
When something takes charge of the beings,
    we speak of the Heart.   25
When the Heart applies itself, we speak of Intent.
When Intent becomes permanent, we speak of Will.
When the persevering Will changes, we speak of Thought.
When Thought extends itself powerfully and far,
    we speak of Reflection.
When Reflection can have all beings at its disposal,
    we speak of Knowing-How.   30

Characters 84 to 186

歧伯答曰
Qi bo da yue

天之在我者德也
tian zhi zai wo zhe de ye

地之在我者氣也
di zhi zai wo zhe qi ye

德流氣薄而生者也
de liu qi bo er sheng zhe ye

故生之來謂之精
gu sheng zhi lai wei zhi jing

兩精相搏謂之神
liang jing xiang bo wei zhi shen

隨神往來者謂之魂
sui shen wang lai zhe wei zhi hun

並精而出入者謂之魄
bing jing er chu ru zhe wei zhi po

所以任物者謂之心
suo yi ren wu zhe wei zhi xin

心有所憶謂之意
xin you suo yi wei zhi yi

意之所存謂之志
yi zhi suo cun wei zhi zhi

因志而存變謂之思
yin zhi er cun bian wei zhi si

因思而遠慕謂之慮
yin si er yuan mu wei zhi lü

因慮而處物謂之智
yin lü er chu wu wei zhi zhi

Heaven within me is Virtue.
Earth within me is Breaths.
Virtue flows down, Breaths expand, and there is life.
  (lines 18, 19, 20)

All life unfolds between Heaven and Earth; the formulation of Heaven/
Earth is the prototype for every living being. Zhang Jiebin's commentary
recalls this, retracing the great features of cosmogenesis, which itself
is biogenesis:

> Man mines the Breaths of Heaven/Earth in order to live.
> Heaven and Earth are ways (routes) of *yin/yang*, *yin yang*
> *zhi dao* 陰陽之道.
>   Out of the Great Ultimate *tai ji* 太極 the two principles
> *er yi* 二儀[13] are produced; thus clear *qing* 清 *yang* produces
> Heaven, and unclear *zhuo* 濁 *yin* produces Earth. Out of the
> two principles the Ten Thousand beings are produced; thus
> *Qian* 乾 (the trigram corresponding to celestial power)
> achieves the great beginning *da shi* 大始, and *Kun* 坤 (the
> trigram corresponding to terrestrial power) accomplishes
> *cheng* 成 all beings.
>   Hence the *Yijing* (*Book of Changes*) says: "The great Vir-
> tue *da de* 大德 of Heaven/Earth is called life (or the living,
> *sheng* 生)."
>   And Chapter 25 of the *Suwen*: "Man lives on Earth, and
> his destiny *ming* 命 hangs *xuan* 懸 from Heaven."
>   Thus *yang* is first (*xian* 先) and *yin* comes after (*hou* 後).
> *Yang* diffuses and *yin* receives.
>   The Virtue that opens into life is rooted in Heaven. The
> breaths through which forms are accomplished are rooted
> *ben* in Earth. Therefore, within me, Heaven is Virtue and
> Earth is Breaths. Virtue flows down, the Breaths expand,
> and life *is*. In this complete and natural way, forms are
> produced and accomplished.

Writers of antiquity, whose names have not survived but who were
the first to enclose the doctrine of needles in the classical text, connected
all living beings to the Virtue of Heaven and the Breaths of Earth.

---

[13] The *yin* and the *yang*.

Normally everything we live with under Heaven is the outpouring of the heavenly Virtue; streaming down upon us is the gift that never runs dry. Our heart beats in response to the life that is offered to it. We call it Virtue and attribute it definitively to Heaven. The existence of "I" *wo* 我 is Virtue expressed. The Virtue of Heaven, or simply Virtue, is always the Virtue of the Way *dao de* 道德. We know that this Way is Heaven's Virtue.

Covered and incubated by Heaven, we surge into being and come to life. The gift is renewed. If it were no longer to be granted, the life that we know would cease to exist within us, as would the life in all living beings. Later in this text we shall consult the commentators to clarify and expand upon what the Virtue of Heaven is that constitutes myself within me.

Normally Virtue is placed in dependence on the heart within a Being. The heart shelters Heaven. Illuminated by Heaven's radiance and by the Spirits, the heart is able to recognize the correctness and the authenticity of conduct. Why? Because Heaven within us is our virtue, just as outside us Heaven is the Virtue of all virtue.

Virtue is the mooring of life in Heaven. Coming from Heaven it gives true nature, natural principles, development, and authenticity. The presence of Heaven within me creates the way for finding my natural or heavenly tendencies *li* 理. All schools of Chinese thought are in agreement on this point. The commentators attest to it:

> Virtue is obtained *de* 得 from Heaven which is empty, filled with marvelous impulses, and without darkness; the entire ensemble of norms *li* 理[14] resonates *ying* 應,[15] with the Ten Thousand human affairs.
>
> *Zhang Zhicong*

> It is not that Heaven does not have breaths, but it has the mastery *zhu* 主 to give the natural tendencies (or norms) *li*. Thus the virtue that is in me is the Virtue of Heaven.
>
> *Ma Shi*

What is received from Heaven is marked indelibly, actively, and constantly. All conduct proceeds from there. Under this provenance are the conduct of the person, and the conduct of the acupuncturist working

---

[14] Natural arrangements.
[15] In correspondence.

to restore life. The pathways of the meridians in us are an image of the correctness and constancy taken by animation and form, responding to the impetus of Virtue from Heaven. However, form and animation can only appear through actions appropriate to Earth.

Spirits are of the same nature as the Virtue of Heaven in us, and they are also its messengers. Virtue, like the Spirits, is luminous radiance *ming* 明 . It is the "Light that lights all things coming into this world" (Gospel of John, 1:9). The Spirits, filled with light, rush to us and arrive in us. Virtue is brought by them and manifested in us.

In the coupling of Way/Virtue *dao/de*, Virtue follows the Way like a lady-in-waiting; Virtue itself is the effective, beneficent pouring out, the spreading out, the impulse, the source that forms the inspiration for conduct. Heaven is manifested by Virtue, which then naturally flows down from on high. Laozi is speaking of the flowing down of Virtue when he says in the *Daodejing*, Chapter 8:

> Good descends from On High like water.

The creative movement of Heaven is considered the immeasurable *yang*, the limitless height and profusion of vivifying power that is released effortlessly. This supreme *yang* holds within itself a "seed" of *yin*. Because of this its impulses can descend, touch, penetrate and enliven the Earth.

Chapter 5 of the *Suwen* shows the movements of clouds and rain. The movements we call physiological are analogous repetitions of these movements, particularly the exchanges among the *zang* inside the torso. In this way they are shown to be efficient and necessary.

Qi Bo's response gives thirteen propositions. Virtue holds the first place, at the level of the symbolic meaning of the number One. Virtue, accompanied by the going and coming of the Spirits that bring it to us, remains the guarantee of unity, of the cohesion and stability of the luminous progression. Virtue attests to the power of Heaven in man. Virtue is the "follower" of the Way, and the Spirits are its escort.

Light, reason, Great Reason *da li* 大理 — to use the expression of the philosopher Xunzi — confers nobility and guarantees correct and righteous living. Authenticity is the very substance of the rectitude of living beings; it is a faithfulness to oneself because of the excellence of Heaven operating within us. The Way of Heaven leads us in all our ways. At the moment when it is acting in us, it is right to speak of Virtue.

Morality is at the center of the notion of *de*, Virtue. The conduct of life proceeds from that which is received and assimilated and from the manner in which the sorting and eliminating are handled. It is a matter of physical or mental exercise, moral conduct, and vigilant attention to all the physical and psychic balancings. It is merely a question of knowing how to lead one's life, to bring it closer to its true nature, and to avoid all waste and all conflict that has no real significance. One seeks the greatest possible longevity, within the definite limits of one's species.

Qi Bo's answer will lead to knowing, the knowing-how-to-live from which proceeds Long Life. It is rooted in virtue and in the way in which each being is capable of receiving, accepting, and enlightening it, in order to restore one's own natural light.

> Our body can be produced only by the *dao*, and our life can shine only through Virtue *de*. One who conserves life and reaches the fullness of his days is one who — upon the foundation of Virtue — has caused the Way *dao* to gleam. Isn't that the Royal Virtue *wang de* 王德 ? Majestically one emerges from the Indistinct; he advances full of power, and the Ten Thousand beings follow in his wake.
>
> *Zhuangzi*, Chapter 12

Only he who has found himself, who possesses himself and possesses virtue, is fit to govern.

The Breaths of Earth

The Chinese conception speaks of Heaven only in opposition to, in contrast with, and as complementing and co-penetrating Earth. Once it is established that Heaven within me is Virtue and determines Level One, then Earth within me is that which carries and receives this Virtue and gives it forever-evolving forms.

For — and this may be startling — form is not the only way to show Earth's welcome of the celestial impulse authored by Heaven. Earth is the great purveyor of forms, in which the gifts from Heaven are lodged. But even before speaking of forms *xing* 形 , we must introduce the form-without-specific-form, that which bends itself to become all forms: the Breaths *qi* 氣 .

Earth within me is Breaths. Let us dwell for a moment on this remarkable fact: that the only true form that is opposable, contrasting, complementary to and co-penetrable by the immense Virtue of Heaven, is the form of all things — Breath.

The character *qi* used in the singular, "Breath," indicates a large meaning that avoids the effect of abstract generalities. Used in the plural, "Breaths," it helps us understand that in a concrete being it is responsible for the constitution and the animation of the being. Whether we say Breath or Breaths, it is always a matter of a co-penetration and a *yin/yang* exchange.

With Earth, we are at the level of the symbolic meaning of the number Two. The diversity and diversification appropriate to Earth are expressed in the fact that the breaths are *yin* and *yang*; they are also *yin/yang*. The breaths must not be qualified as *yang*. Breaths are the concrete relation between the two poles of *yin* and *yang*; the breaths are the exchanges between them.

It may be surprising to see the breaths *qi* characterizing Earth, when it is said in other circumstances that breaths belong to Heaven. But what characterizes Heaven even more than breaths, is Unity, the norm of each existence, of each living being. This unity is expressed as the Virtue of the Breaths, whereas Earth is characterized as The Breaths of Virtue. Earth possesses virtue, but virtue is not the specific terrestrial effect felt within me. Let us turn now to a good commentator:

> It is not that Earth does not have Virtue, but it has the distribution *yun* 運 of Breaths *qi*; thus the Breaths that are in me are the Breaths of Earth.
>
> *Ma Shi*

If the aspect of norm and correctness is attributed to Heaven under the name of Virtue, Earth will claim Breaths for its own account by emphasizing the duality of *yin/yang* (the multiplicity of their movements, and of the forms they generate). Earth permits the junctions and regulations, and the effective distribution of differentiated breaths. All the transformations that affect forms, between their moment of appearance and moment of disappearance, are held within Earth's bosom. And all of this takes place under Heaven's incitement, permitting the appropriate operations within a particular being:

The vision of the eye, the hearing of the ear, the odors of the nose, the tastes of the mouth, the manipulations of the hand, the steps of the feet – all of this is produced on Earth by the forms/breaths *xing qi* 形氣 .

Zhang Zhicong

Within me this power is the Beaths, the varied aspects of my animation, of my corporeal and mental being. Earth, in me, is the presence of diversity, of varied and multiple aspects, under the authority of the celestial unity that forges a being. It is also the ceaseless transformations.

The breaths extend everywhere; they occupy available space without encumbering it; they are light and fluid, which permits their junction and co-penetrations and also their rising to meet Heaven. The breaths of Earth are not imprisoned; all they ask is to intersect each other under the impulse of Heaven.

Thus all that is breaths in me is Earth, breaths projected toward the one Heaven. For Heaven makes these breaths those of one particular being, with its own destiny and nature.

Yin and *yang* form a harmonized Breath *he qi* 和氣, substance *zhi* 質 accomplishes my being, and it is the Way of Earth *di zhi dao* 地之道 .

The division within the heart of Virtue causes flowing and movement *liu dong* 流動; the *yin/yang* Breaths are harmonized and established; that which brings about a division within the Formless *wu xing* 無形 is appropriate to the Way of Heaven *tian zhi dao* 天之道 .

The Breaths in movement are harmonized and established, and life is conferred upon beings *wu de sheng* 物得生.

Taisu

This passage is largely inspired by Chapter 12 of *Zhuangzi*. There are good translations available for reference.

The Junction of Life

At the level of the symbolic meaning of Three, we have life, the living, the vital thrust *sheng* 生 . This life is the result of a crossing. There is no life, nor are there living beings, except through the *yin/yang* breaths, submissive to Earth's appropriate action and individuated by Heaven.

Life weaves its way through the norm, structure, and vigor given by Heaven, and through the Breaths continually provided by Earth. Life is the result of an exchange that is maintained continually in me.

In Chapter 42 Laozi goes from that place of junction, from the impulse of the level of Three, directly to the Ten Thousand things, to the totality of the living. Chapter 8 of the *Lingshu* deals with a man's own life (hence the expression "within me"). We shall, therefore, lay out the sequence of the above proceedings appropriate to man from the moment of the vital meeting.

The ideogram *sheng*, life, shows how every living thing — be it plant or man (see Glossary at Life) — has the virtue and the uprightness necessary to raise it toward Heaven, displaying its "antlers" to the right and the left, while remaining rooted, and drawing upon its multiple resources from Earth.

The level of these three propositions (Virtue, Breaths, Life) is both cosmic and human. Man exists and subsists only at the junction of Heaven and Earth.

As for the relationship between life *sheng* and transformations *hua* 化, Earth is the support for the transformations that produce life, that form life, and that are life. The *Book of Changes* illustrates this profound certitude of Chinese thought.

The coming forth of living beings indicates the Essences.
(line 21)

This is the fourth proposition of Qi Bo's answer, and the fourth level of life (at the symbolic level of the number Four). In the lightning-swift manner of the *Neijing*, this assertion sets forth the origin of living beings and the nature of the essences. If we are more dazzled than enlightened, it is undoubtedly because we are not all initiates! Therefore, we must modestly and patiently go over the three main characters in this line of Qi Bo's response, in order to seize the significance of their sequence and to seek the deep meaning in the commentaries.

生   *Sheng*:   this could be life. In reality, it is the populace of living beings, usually called the Ten Thousand Beings, under Heaven.

來   *Lai*:   the Ten Thousand Beings rush forth; they appear like the springtime that takes us by surprise by arriving suddenly.

精   *Jing*:   the Essences.

Living beings come forth; they emerge from their Essences. We shall see that the Essences *jing* form a grouping that reunites the determining aspects of the species (particularized into varieties and/or individuals), establishes the individual being, presides over its development, its preservation, and its identity, permits its autonomy, and furthers its affinity and assimilation within certain constraints of compatibility.

The Essences themselves are not visible. But living beings emerge from their mass and mark an instance where the particular origin and the specific nature of a being are joined to create that being. One who takes the trouble can perceive and observe the presence of differentiated lives within the bosom of the One. It is not our purpose to reduce the mystery of the existence of the many beings living diversely in the universal flow.

An objective description of a Being will find that the Being is faithful to its nature. One can count on its fidelity for the simple reason that it exists and subsists only as "authentic Virtue." Where there is purity there is perfect development from the essences.

We can count on the fidelity of beings, but we must also reckon with it. See, for example, the behavior of monkey-keepers (*Zhuangzi*, Chapter 2) and tamers of tigers (*Zhuangzi*, Chapter 4). Knowing the capricious nature of monkeys and the carnivorous fury of tigers when excited by blood, their keepers feed and care for each according to the precautions imposed by their natures.

Life would not be possible within the community of the living without fidelity to the Essences that specifically establish the being of Beings. A reading of texts of the Daoist tradition (*Laozi*, Chapters 6, 21, 42 and 55, and *Zhuangzi*, Chapters 2, 11, 12, 15, 17, 19, 22 and 25) shows that this doctrine is identical everywhere and is expressed in a vocabulary that must be patiently identified and always respected. Qi Bo's formula, "The coming forth of living beings indicates the Essences," is the very expression of the movement from consideration of the Breath of life (the web of life that is forever being spun [*Laozi*, Chapter 6]), to consideration of the "Ten Thousand Breaths that are each different," (*Zhuangzi*, Chapter 2). Laozi, in Chapters 21 and 42, corroborates this way of seeing.

Let us recapitulate the first four affirmations of Qi Bo's answer:

The complex unity of life is perceived through contemplation of the Virtue of Heaven and consideration of the Breaths of Earth, both of which are co-penetrated by each other. We shall call "Life" this co-penetration whereby the breaths refer me back to Virtue, just as Virtue refers me back to the breaths. Living beings come and show themselves in Ten Thousand ways. Struck by the different aspects and forms, I question myself as to the origins of the Ten Thousand Beings. As I am sensitive to their common origin and yet do not want to ignore their original differences, I must find a word. Essences *jing* is the one that fits.

The essences reveal themselves as the natural movement of life. Life produces itself, is produced, appears, embellishes itself, spreads out and expands itself in a deep cooperation with the essences. Life and each living being are always in a process of conjoining and reunion.

> By itself, *yin* cannot produce *sheng*; by itself, *yang* cannot produce; by itself, Heaven cannot produce. But from the conjoining of these three *san he* 三合 , life flows out naturally *ran hou sheng* 然後生.
>
> *Yijing*

This reunion of three is, in fact, Heaven inseminating the terrestrial *yin/yang*. There must always be a joining to create life, to create a living being. Therefore, the essences are the power derived from conjoining. The essences take what is available to them: either another complementary essence in equally pure form, or any other materials for the renewal of a being. From these they then form the basis of life. The essences are concentration, assimilation, and marvelous reliability that guarantee unity and authenticity. They recompose this unity and authenticity by sorting, choosing, accepting and rejecting in order to assimilate.

The Essences are the root *ben* 本 of Being.

> *Suwen*, Chapter 4

Chapter 49, *"Neiye,"* of *Guanzi* speaks of the rooting of all that exists in the world:

> The Essences in all beings are what make them alive. Below, they produce the five cereals (grains). Above, they create the stars and arrange them in order. They flow *liu* 流 into the space of Heaven/Earth and we call this the Spirits

of Earth and of Heaven *gui shen* 鬼神 . When they are stored *cang* 藏 in the middle of the chest, we call the person who stores them a holy man *sheng ren* 聖人 . Thus are the breaths. . . .

Whatever exists, exists through and with the essences. Specifically, they give the characteristics of the species that animate each being. One could be tempted by "genetic engineering," by the manipulation of Essences, to modify —theoretically improving — that which comprises and recomposes itself spontaneously. This question had already caused torment in *Zhuangzi*:

> The General of the clouds said: "The breaths of Heaven being without harmony *he* 和 , the breaths of Earth being smothered, the Six Breaths being in disorder, the order of the Four Seasons being irregular, I would like to re-make the joining of the essences of the Six Breaths to insure maintenance of the numberless numbers of the living. What must I do?"
>
> *Zhuangzi*, Chapter 11

The only answer is: do not be concerned with that; instead seek natural conduct.

We do not change the givens of life. The essences make life specific at the core of the universal vitality. They regulate the conditions of life for each being from birth to death, from appearance to disappearance. Heaven/Earth, the expression of Nature, knows innately how to utilize the essences. Man, in imitating Heaven/Earth, learns to maintain himself in his being, harmonizing his constituent parts, opportunely storing his reserves, avoiding wasting his natural resources, giving out when he should shed something, and holding in when he should preserve something. From this knowledge of maintenance evolve techniques for breathing, diet, meditation, and sexual hygiene — techniques that should be called "essential."

Hidden though the essences may be, they are not inaccessible. They show in a person's appearance and shape and in the revelation from inside to outside that can be known through minute and intense observation. The essences allow themselves to be seen in the natural being who does not hide what creates him (cf. *Laozi*, Chapter 21).

We can ascertain a person's nature and the variable state of that person's nature as functions of the moment, of the season, of time, and of traces left by life on the body. We can also discern it in the language and the manner of the person. But the perception is after all only conjecture. One might be tempted to abuse this perception and become manipulative. Analysis can reveal the composition of a being, but it stops short of revealing the movement that brings the being into life and that allows him to leave in the same way he has come.

There is no access to the nonmanifest, to the root of beings, if by access we mean a way that can penetrate into beings. The essences belong to the category of "secret wonders," of which Laozi speaks (Chapter 1). A "wonder" is not an object for consideration. It is the forever-hidden face of all beings. It is good to contemplate this "Way," of which it is said:

> One looks in vain; there is nothing to see.
>
> *Laozi*, Chapter 35

What is called (later in Chinese history) the essences of Anterior Heaven, is the first composition of a particular being. This primary composition does not pre-exist in any way; only the elements of its composition exist. In the life of beings, everything is always related to their primary composition. We can only grasp the ways in which the "authorities" participate in the perpetual re-composition of that particular being.

> Always that which comes first *xian* 先 [16] in the life of a being, is called the essences.
>
> *Lingshu*, Chapter 30

Zhang Zhicong is more precise: it is a matter of the essences received in the first place (anteriorly), from the One Heaven that gives rise to and guarantees the unity of each living being. This occurs before the development and completion of the body. Little by little the body draws out its form from the work of the essences, permitting (through the transformations) the releasing of the breaths and the constitution of all the proceedings. Everything is formed by the essences.

> First of all at the beginning of man's life, the essences compose him perfectly *jing cheng* 精成.
>
> *Lingshu*, Chapter 10

---

[16] Anteriorly. Many texts contain references to Anterior Heaven *xian tian* and Posterior Heaven *hou tian*. Anterior Heaven represents innate energies (genetic and hereditary, given to a new life at the moment of conception), and Posterior Heaven represents acquired energies (the transformation of nutritive energies by the body).

Next come the constitution and completion of the brain, the marrows, the bones, the vessels, the muscles, the flesh, and the layers of skin. Then comes the direct process of renewal when after his birth, the individual dips into his environment to find the wherewithal to re-create his liveliness.

Innateness, nature, is at work from conception to death. The current meaning of the expression, "life comes" *sheng lai* 生來 , is innateness: that which is there from the beginning of life, that which comes with life. When the composition arrives at full term, when the dynamic tension is exhausted along with the decline of *yang*, there is decomposition, a synonym for death.

Thus the essences, resulting from the union of Heaven and Earth, procreate beings through this movement of unison. The existence of a living being is proof that there has been an essential conjoining – a composition of essences.

Though they habitually live upon the side of *yin*, of water, the essences are *yang* essences as well as *yin* essences. There are essences of Heaven, of Earth, of Water, of Fire. Thus in Chapter 3 of the *Suwen* we speak of the essences of *yang* breaths for the maintenance of the Spirits. In Speaking of Heaven/Earth:

> The essences, doubled in harmony, are the *yin/yang*.
> *Huainanzi*, Chapter 3

> When the Great Ultimate *tai ji* 太極 begins movement *dong* 動 , *yang* is produced *sheng yang* 生陽; when it comes to rest *jing* 靜, *yin* is produced *sheng yin* 生陰. Each of the two *yin/yang* breaths has its essences. These essences are the One of Heaven and the Six of Earth. Heaven, through the One, produces water. Earth, through the Six, completes water, and this water is the very first of the Five Elements. That is why water arises at the very beginning of the creation of the Ten Thousand Beings.
>
> *Zhang Jiebin*

Virtue is "the Good that flows from On High like water" (*Laozi*, Chapter 8), the celestial unity pouring itself into each being. The essences represent the flow of life for the ensemble of living beings, and for each particular living being. Through their power of composition, decomposition, and re-composition, the essences form the specific bases for each of the One Hundred Species and for each of the Ten Thousand Beings.

The embrace of the two Essences indicates the Spirits.
   (line 22)

To embrace, carried by a powerful natural desire, is to create a situation so intimate that two Essences give birth to One from their coupling. The two that unite form a pair and mate together; this is the meaning of *liang* 兩 (couple, two of something), as opposed to the meaning of *er* 二 (the number two). The use of "two" (*er*) does not exclude the existence of a couple, but it does not necessarily include it and does not allow a clear understanding of the intimacy of the possible union.

The first couple is formed by the essences of Heaven uniting with the essences of Earth. *All* other couplings reproduce this image. *Yin/yang* is the unitary expression of the binary power of Heaven/Earth. After this all the other couplings come in gradations: water and fire, rooster and hen, and so on.

When speaking of man, in referring to the union of his parents we mean the conjoining of all these coupled movements that are contained in the co-penetration of the breaths of Earth by the Virtue of Heaven. The parents mutually offer what they essentially are: their essences. A new composition results from the joining of the essences of the father with those of the mother. It is this that brings about the arrival of the Spirits.

> Man and woman unite their essences: the Ten Thousand Beings are produced through transformations *hua shen* 化生 .
>
> *Yijing, Xici*

Zhang Jiebin develops the theme in a similar way:

> The *Dao* (the Way) of the production and completion of the Ten Thousand Beings: it is exclusively the *yin/yang* exchange *jiao* 交 and then the luminous radiance of the Spirits *shen ming* 神明 . That is why, to have human life, it is necessary to have a joining of the *yin* and *yang* breaths, a union of the essences of the father and mother. Two essences embrace: (corporeal) form and Spirits are achieved; it is the reunited breaths of Heaven/Earth, and the natural name is man.

A being arises, and the Spirits represent the unity of this living being, as stated in Chapter 15 of the *Suwen*:

The Way is in the unity, and the Spirits *shen* imprint a rotating movement without ever bringing up the rear. If they were in the rear they would no longer guarantee the rotations; the subtle mechanism (of life) *ji* 機 would be lost *shi* 失."

This is illustrated in the Funeral Banner from Tomb 1 at Mawangdui. In the center of the top band of the banner two spirits are mounted on horses that circle as if in a riding ring. They imprint on the Blessed Isles of the East a rotating movement, a spin that they themselves turn in their saddles to watch. The subtle movement of life that guarantees stability through a rotating movement is shown clearly.

The essences are a composite unit, permitting the model for recomposition. The Spirits are the absolute unity, a given. The latter are not *yin/yang* co-mingled; they are beyond any *yin/yang* determination. The Spirits are thus the guarantee of the rotation that assures life, and the effectiveness of its subtle mechanism. This is affirmed in the *Yijing*, and repeated in the *Suwen*.

> Whatever cannot be probed by *yin/yang* is the Spirits.
>
> *Suwen*, Chapter 66

The Spirits alone permit access to true knowledge, to perception of the intimate nature, and of the natural and celestial tendencies of beings and things.

> Perceiving *zhi* 知(knowing) the *Dao* of changes and transformations *bian hua* 變化 is how one perceives the Spirits.
>
> *Yijing*

> When we speak of transformations *hua* and of changes *bian*, it is the free communications going as far as fusion *tong* 通 with the natural, intimate tendencies *li* 理 of the *shen ming*, which is the luminous radiance of the Spirits.
>
> *Suwen*, Chapter 69

Through the Spirits man is capable of truly perceiving his experience, and of relating all phenomena to *yin/yang* (cf. *Suwen*, Chapter 5).

The Spirits draw this power from the fact that they emanate from the original mystery and represent this undifferentiated fusion of all origins (and of each specific origin) in man. Zhang Jiebin affirms that the Spirits in question here can only be qualified as original, *yuan* 元 . The Spirits are the intimate link to the original unity.

The mystery *xuan* 玄 (the profound mystery, which is the original mystery) produces *sheng* the Spirits *shen*.

Suwen, Chapter 5

Like the essences, the Spirits themselves cannot be grasped, and they are the root of all that *can* be grasped. They can only be perceived as support for the visible.

> The Spirits, Oh! the Spirits! The ear cannot hear them, but the heart opens through the brilliance of the eye, and the will is the first to appear. Only penetrating intelligence can understand this. The mouth cannot express it in words; it can only be seen. But it is a chaotic confusion *hun* 混 ; only the bright flash can provoke the radiance; it is like a wind blowing the clouds. This is called the Spirits.
>
> *Suwen*, Chapter 26

The spiritual light, especially that shining in the eyes, reveals our Spirits. These Spirits are first in the heart, in the emptiness of the heart which is their peaceful, tranquil, and unencumbered dwelling place; thus the heart stores the Spirits; the bright radiance of the Spirits *shen ming* emanates from the heart. In Chapter 9 of the *Suwen* it is said:

> The Heart is the rooting of life *sheng zhi ben* 生之本 , the place where changes are made by the Spirits.

The Spirits radiate out from the heart to the smallest nooks and crannies of a being. They are everywhere – in the *zang* 臟 , in the mind, wherever the life force shows.

> The Supreme *Dao*: the Spirits are present at Niwan (upper Field of Cinnabar), as in the One Hundred pathways of animation.
>
> *Huangtingjing*

Omnipresent through all the relays of life and with all imaginable messengers, the Spirits guide life, giving it its deep orientation which is to follow its nature and Nature, and to fulfill a particular vital destiny, a "mandate."

> The Heart is Sovereign and Master of the whole body; Ten Thousand Spirits are at the call of the mandate of life *sheng ming* 生命 . Therefore, the beneficent impulses received in

emptiness bring perception and feelings, sometimes enlivening, sometimes annihilating. According to circumstances,
the [subtle] mechanism [of life] is adapted to situations of a
thousand changes and ten thousand transformations, a thousand *li* in the blink of an eye, a hundred events in the space
of a dream. One can foresee what has not yet occurred; one
can guess good and bad fortune. Big, it is the empire under
Heaven. Small, it is a hairline crack. Nothing else knows
such extremes. As the Spirits are supreme *zhi* 至 (absolute), the heart inevitably is also. When the heart stops, the
Spirits also stop.

> *Jindan dayao*, cited by Zhang Jiebin

The presence of the Spirits is life; their departure is death. This
formula is repeated many times throughout the *Neijing* in diverse
forms:

> If the Spirits leave us, there is death.
>
> *Lingshu*, Chapter 71

> Possession of the Spirits *de shen* 得神 is the splendor
> *chang* 昌 of life; loss of the Spirits *shi shen* 失神 is ruin
> *wang* 亡 .
>
> *Suwen*, Chapter 13

We can easily understand that nothing equals the Spirits, that there
is nothing more valuable than being anchored in, or moored by, the
Spirits. We must take vigilant care for the guarding of the Spirits *shou
shen* 守神 and allow them to lead our life, without opposing them.
All opposition necessarily reveals a perversion of nature and, in time,
exhaustion of the natural being, as for example an exhaustion of one's
essences leading irrevocably to the loss of the Spirits, and thus of life.
Zhang Jiebin may conclude:

> When the Spirits are overwhelmed, they leave; when left
> in peace, they remain. Thus the most important thing in the
> conduct and treatment of a being is maintenance of the
> Spirits *yang shen* 養神 , and then comes maintenance of
> the body *yang xing* 養形 .

To maintain the Spirits is to arrange their stay in a heart that is
peaceable and empty. Rules of moral and passionate life help those who
believe that nothing is more important than the Spirits and the storing

of Essences that establishes their dwelling-place. We find rules of dietetics, sexual conduct, and physical exercise to reinforce, in every way, the essences that serve us from within to sustain and welcome the Spirits (cf. *Laozi*, Chapter 28).

We must know how to behave like a hen as well as a rooster, conserving the *yin/yang* balance, in order to maintain powerful Spirits in a healthy body.

The successful co-penetration of the essences of the father and the mother are at the origin of the arising of a new being, calling the Spirits to come. They are present and they guard the essences. Such is the primordial state. All that remains is to support it according to the model given by the essences. According to a later vocabulary than that of the *Neijing*, it is also a matter of the perpetually successful conjoining of the essences said to be from Anterior Heaven, with the essences said to be from Posterior Heaven. These two essences embrace and form only one, "my" vital essence, which is the basis for releasing the breaths and the varied aspects of "my" being. Thus there is nothing to trouble the Spirits or to prevent them from communicating the Way of Life. This is the interpenetration spoken of by Zhang Zhicong:

> The *Lingshu*, Chapter 32, says: "The Spirits are the essences/breaths *jing/qi* of the liquids and grains." There are the essences of life rooted in Anterior Heaven, and the essences of the liquids and cereals of Posterior Heaven (whose work is to vitalize), and now here are the Spirits! That is why it is said that when the two essences embrace, it indicates the Spirits.

The indissoluble bond of the essences and the Spirits leads us to stop at the idea of essences/Spirits *jing/shen*, contenting ourselves to give several quotations without analysis or commentary.

> The *jing shen* of the Saints *sheng ren* 聖人 would not be dispersed.
>
> *Suwen*, Chapter 1

> The authentic men of High Antiquity . . .exhale and inhale the essences/breaths *jing qi*; they guard the Spirits *shou shen* 守神 , being well established in themselves.
>
> *Suwen*, Chapter 1

If the *yin* are spread out and the *yang* tightly condensed, essences/Spirits *jing shen* govern themselves as they should *zhi* 治 .

Suwen, Chapter 3

The blood and breaths *xue qi*, and the essences and Spirits *jing shen*, of man offer life and fulfill perfectly the natural destiny *xing ming* 性命 of each.

Lingshu, Chapter 47

Huangdi said: "The *zang* 臟 store *cang* 藏 the essences and the Spirits *jing shen* and the *hun* 魂 and the *po* 魄. The *fu* 腑 offer the liquids and the cereals as well as their transformations and their circulation in the form of material."

Lingshu, Chapter 52

Mawangdui Funeral Banner (next page): This painting on silk, discovered in a tomb from the 2nd century B.C., shows the human destiny after death. At the top (A) is the Paradise of peace and equilibrium, into which the soul of the deceased hopes to merge. Here is the axis that distributes the flowing movements making living beings though the play of yin *and* yang *(represented by two dragons). In the middle (B), two individuals greet the deceased on her journey toward Heaven; she is followed by her three Hun souls. Farther down (C), a funeral banquet is being arranged around the casket of the deceased. Seven individuals symbolize the Po souls. Their task is to return into the depths of Earth what belongs there.*

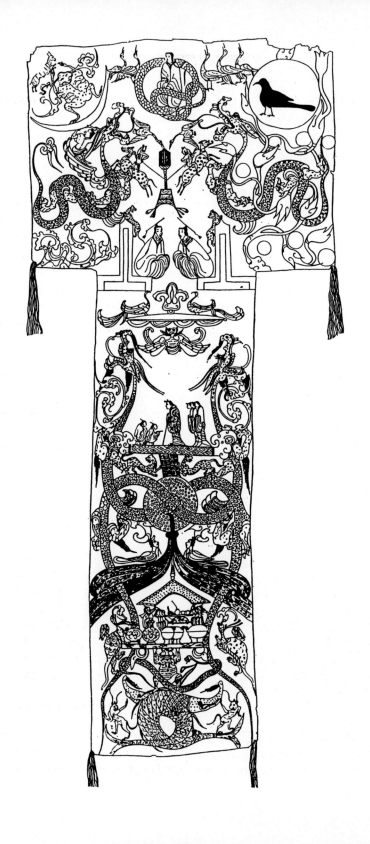

*That which follows the Spirits faithfully in their going and
coming indicates the **Hun**.*
*That which associates with the Essences in their exiting
and entering indicates the **Po**. (lines 23, 24)*

Tradition commonly gives to the *Hun* the *yang* aspect of the Spirits,
expressed by the *yang* breaths that are subtle, light, and airy. The *Po*
are given the *yin* aspect of the Spirits, expressed by the *yin* essences
that are less subtle, less light, more earthly. By their firmness these
latter are apt to grasp specifically and concretely the impulse coming
from the Spirits.

The three *Hun* and the seven *Po* are represented on the Mawangdui
Banner (Tomb 1). The *Hun* accompany the deceased princess, marching behind her into emptiness, sliding more than marching, the hem
of their robes caught in a whirlwind. The *Po*, lower down, are immobile,
in a receptive attitude, close to the ground or in contact with it, among
the ritual vases containing the essences of grain and fermented drinks.
Hun and *Po* are in the service of the princess whose colors they carry.
The *Hun* are in charge of her immortal destiny, and the *Po* are busy
with more domestic tasks. The numbers – three for the *Hun* and seven
for the *Po* – are perfectly suited for bringing the *Hun* closer to Heaven
and taking the *Po* from life to the dissolution that is their destined end.

A commentator explains how the Spirits, being *yang* as opposed to
the essences, can themselves be further discerned as *yin* and *yang*,
declaring the *Po yin* and the *Hun yang*:

> When we contrast essences with Spirits, the Spirits are
> *yang* and the essences are *yin*. When we contrast the *Hun*
> and *Po,* the *Hun* are *yang* and the *Po* are *yin*. Thus the *Hun*
> faithfully follow the Spirits in their going and coming, and
> the *Po* are associated with the essences in their entering and
> exiting. . . .The Spirits are *yang* within the *yang*; the *Hun* are
> *yin* within the *yang*; the essences are *yin* within *yin*; the *Po*
> are *yang* within *yin*. By correctly distinguishing *yin* and
> *yang*, and determining the authenticity of the *Hun* and *Po*,
> one can go to the limits of dreams.
>
> *Zhang Jiebin*

We see the relativity of *yin/yang* distinctions according to the couplings where they appear. Thus the Spirits, by themselves, are above
all *yin/yang* determinations; however, this will not prevent their being

called *yang* when they appear in a coupling with the essences. It will also not prevent our seeing in the *Hun* the expression of *yang* that is in the Spirits, nor in the *Po* what there is of *yin* in the Spirits.

The *Hun* – *yang* movement – tend to rise to the heights. At death, they become in Heaven the glorious spirits of the dead. During life, they lift themselves in intelligence, knowledge, sensitivity, spirituality, and imagination. But to do this they must be rooted in the *yin* to hold them firmly, preventing the fatal accomplishment of their flight toward Heaven. They are stored by the Liver and thus rooted in the *yin*. The Liver is a male *zang*, an outlet for the strong effects of *yang*, but it has its origin in the Kidneys (essences and marrows of the Kidneys). The Liver has a profoundly *yin* nature; it is the great storehouse, the keeper of the blood. This blood makes an ideal dwelling-place for the *Hun*, allowing them a place to alight, as birds from the sky are offered a nest or a perch. In reciprocity, the *Hun* bestow a spiritual quality to the blood.

The *Po*, whose movement is *Yin*, tend to bury themselves in the depths. At death, they return to the earth whose richness they renew in the process of slowly decomposing and disappearing.

> Flesh and bones are buried and become like the soil of the fields.
>
> *Liji*, Couvreur translation, II, p. 289

During the course of life the *Po* are responsible for our vital movements, our sensations, our reactions, and our instinctive thrusts. All that is sensory, "vegetative," and corporeal is obedient to them. They depend on their solid rooting in the *yang*. This sustains them, completes and harmonizes them, and prevents their fatal return to Earth, into the earth. Thus the lungs store the *Po*. The Lung is a female *zang*; it gathers in breaths and Spirits, like the season of autumn. It is also the master of the breaths, and in particular it has the charge of the cyclic regulations, or the instinctive rhythms of life. The breaths are the support of the *Po*, allowing them to express themselves in animating the being.

Let us move to the difference in the formulas that bind the *Hun* to Spirits *shen* and the *Po* to essences *jing*.

Going and coming *wang lai* 往來 characterizes Spirits. Going and coming, circulating freely, maintaining relationships and subtle exchanges, all of these together weave life on the cosmic loom.

> Limitless going and coming is called free communication *tong* 通.
>
> *Yijing, Xici*

The reality of my life is the going and coming of the Spirits. They alone are capable of reaching all the way to the deep natural tendencies. Spirits see Spirits and speak to Spirits. They alone have the capacity to speak to me of me, to help me meet others deeply and intimately. The *Hun* enjoy the freedom of the Spirits. They guarantee the exchanges that lead us to reality and to the avoidance of delirium, perversion, and aberration.

We suggest a re-reading of *Zhuangzi*, Chapter 2. The *Hun* are spoken of there. During sleep they make connections and relationships. These are different from the difficulties we have communicating during our waking hours, where we hurl ourselves at the multiplicity of limits that other beings set to render themselves opaque. What a difference between that and the intimacy the *Hun* develop among themselves during sleep! To be more concrete, it suffices to remember what we said about the lightness and the subtle capacity of Spirits to come in noiselessly and to leave us without our knowledge. This marvelous faculty of penetration and of spiritual intelligence also belongs to the *Hun*, which faithfully follow the Spirits in their movements. There is this difference: the *Hun* are ours absolutely; the Spirits are of Heaven and are its messengers to us.

> Confucius was thinking of that when he sighed: "Ah! How many times have I already seen the Duke of Zhou in my dreams!"

The Duke of Zhou, one of the founders of the Zhou dynasty, died several centuries before Confucius. Confucius's dream must have been an authentic meeting of his *Hun* with the spirits of the Duke. Our dreams are communion with the reality that creates us and holds us. When a dream loses its way, it must be straightened out to avoid the danger of potential disorganization that the dream can either encourage or opportunely call the being away from. For this reason, inspection of dreams belongs to diagnosis and has its place in medicine. One must be watchful to see that the breaths are directed well by the Spirits. Spirits and *Hun* are the pivot of health, more than are the *Po*.

During their goings and comings, travels, excursions and ramblings, and during their flights through space, ecstatically riding the wind, are the Spirits and the *Hun* in the body or outside the body? The question is pointless. Spirits and *Hun* are free of the constraints of Earth. Even so, it is not well for their absence to last too long. The body would suffer, and the *Po*, feeling neglected by the *shen*, would be tempted to return to the nether world, and there would be death.

The going and coming of the Spirits, escorted by the *Hun*, are not a disorderly agitation. They require calm and serenity.

> If the heart can really become like an absolute void *tai xu* 太虛, it will necessarily be clear *qing* 清, and tranquil *jing* 靜, and then dreams will give the sensation of life or of death, and consciousness will be profoundly expanded.
>
> *Zhang Jiebin*

Sharpness of intelligence, finesse of understanding, an enlightened spirit, and a vivacious precision demand the freedom implied in the expression "going and coming" (line 23).

The companionship in this freedom is the natural relationship of the *Hun* to the Spirits. In this way the *Hun* faithfully follow the Spirits and gently conform to the Spirits' inspiration, as the prince's escort freely obeys the prince, or as things ideally stand between a couple, or in a friendly relationship.

In the character *sui* 隨 (to follow faithfully) there is a notion of free will. Of one's free will one conforms to a natural unfolding that fulfills hopes. *Sui* is the seventeenth of the sixty-four hexagrams in the *Book of Changes*, and it is defined thus:

> Conformity and unfolding, the moment when one fits into the universal development.

"Exiting and entering" *chu ru* 出入 (line 24) is something else. The activity is one of relationship, but it is more concrete. Here beings and the composite parts of beings are introduced and rejected, caused to appear and disappear. It is domestic work. It is the accounting of life with its entrances and exits, its recipes and its expenses. We open and close; we hire and we fire.

The first of the exits is the exit into the world, the moment of conception or birth, like the plant emerging from the soil (the classical etymology of the ideogram *chu* 出, to exit). Conversely, the last of the entrances − burial, the return to earth − is death. This is the return to the undifferentiated state from which the particular form of this living being had earlier emerged. Between these two principal exits and entrances, life weaves itself through a multitude of exitings and enterings: breathing and taking nourishment (with digestion, assimilation and excretion) are the large physical examples, as well as being the two great functions of survival. Beyond this an infinity of enterings and exitings causes the breaths to pass instinctively from the interior to the exterior, then from the outside back to the inside of a being. These breaths are hot or cold as are reactions, stimuli, emotions. All of life's movements obey the *Po*. There is far more pre-determination and far less freedom in the exitings and enterings than there was in the goings and comings.

All the transformations inherent to the operations of life are equally present in these exitings and enterings. Between that which exits and that which enters (or vice versa) are all the processes for capturing the vital elements, to attach and fuse them to the being that receives and ejects. This is the domain of the essences.

There is a natural relationship of association between the essences and the *Po*. *Bing* 並 means to place oneself in a double harness, or to yoke oneself together with another in a double harness. It is no longer a question of one companion following another, but of the two associating intimately to bend themselves to a common task. It is the nature of the essences to act thus. They do not go rambling about; they grasp life. All relationship with them occurs through this grasping. The *yin* power of concentration exists in the *Po* as in the essences. Throughout the transformations, via the exitings and enterings, this power gives all form to a living being. In this way the *Po* are in relationship with the body and with the constituents of the body.

Their faculty of grasping sometimes makes the *Po* dangerous. When a person dies a violent death, the power of his grasp of life is not exhausted. It refuses to melt into the earth; all life passing within reach interests him. Fear of cemeteries and of the nearness of the dead comes from this: their *Po* may still be strong enough to take possession of another life, one that is poorly armed for its own defense, such as that of a young child.

The residual strength of souls does not depend solely upon the brutality of the death, but also on the age of the individual: a young person who dies is more unquenched than an old person. The conditions of the earthly life lived may also affect the tenacity of the *Po*: *Po* who lived richly may remain demanding.

The *Hun*, like the *Po*, are especially vigorous and enlightened, strong and intelligent, since they have benefitted from essences of quality, drawn abundantly from choice substances. A man who eats and drinks in a gastronomically suitable way, who correctly breathes pure air, who nourishes himself with elevated conversations and great music, reinforces in himself the foundation of his spiritual power, of his *Hun* and his *Po*, of his entire instinctive, corporeal and spiritual being. Here we are referring to a passage in the *Spring and Autumn Annals* (the "Chronicle of the Principality of Lou," Vol. III, p. 142). Over the course of life the *Hun* and *Po* are charged with vitality. The quality of what they absorb creates a concrete vitality whose power is not extinguished by the disassociation brought on by death.

The *Hun* and *Po* live as a couple; their union is life, their separation is our death (*Laozi*, Chapter 10). Their joining balances them and causes them to inhabit the being they compose, stabilized by Blood and Breaths. The *Hun* cleave to the *Po* and the *Po* to the *Hun*, interpenetrating each other. The word "embrace" applies here, as it does to all the other couples that "are" life and that "make" life. A weakening of the mutual passion leads, through distancing, to separation and to divorce. Each partner follows its own natural movement: the *Hun* reach the heights of the heavens, and the *Po* leave by the orifices (especially the lower ones) and fall to earth. The *Hun* shine in the heights and the *Po* try to satisfy themselves in the depths. Then the *Hun* and *Po* have disappeared, melted down again in the universal power where all beings are designed.

Thus *Hun* and *Po*, which join together between conception and death to compose an existence, have an afterlife.

Two citations from the *Neijing* allow us to distinguish the roles of the *Hun* and the *Po* and their place in the construction and vital function-ing of a man living in a body.

> The good concentration (and distribution) of the Essences/Spirits operates through the harmonious conjunction *he* 和 of will and intent *zhi yi* 志意, *Hun* and *Po* do not disperse *san* 散 , neither sorrow nor anger arises, and the five *zang* do not receive perverse energy.
>
> *Lingshu*, Chapter 47

> Huangdi asks: "What then are the Spirits *shen*?"
>
> Qi Bo answers: "Blood and Breaths being well harmonized, maintenance and defense *ying/wei* 營衛 being in good com-munication *tong*, the five *zang* having constituted their unity, the Spirits/Breaths *shen*/qi being sheltered in the heart, the *Hun* and the *Po* are in perfect conjunction, and man is pro-duced."
>
> *Lingshu*, Chapter 54

"Continuity within change" characterizes the movement of life. This is precisely what makes the translation of the *Neijing* texts so exacting. Those who risk it are likely to favor continuity at the expense of change, or change at the expense of continuity. In the former case the translated text seems at a standstill, and in the latter there is such a multiplicity of aspects that the movement of life is concealed rather than revealed. If one tried to make a definite assertion at a clearly-marked point of the welling-up or the regular flowing-out of life, it would be impossible to use one single expression or term for that assertion. We shall demonstrate this in the two following excerpts and in our conclusion to this presentation of the *Hun* and the *Po*. Two texts, one from Chapter 23 of the *Suwen* and the other from Chapter 62, show how to establish the correct relationships of affinity between the five *zang* on the one hand, the *Hun* and the *Po* on the other, and also the blood and breaths. First the excerpts:

> This is the treasure stored (thesaurized) by the Five *Zang*: the Heart stores the Spirits; the Lung stores the *Po;* the Liver stores the *Hun*, the Spleen stores the Intent *yi* 意 ; the Kidneys store the Will *zhi* 志 . These are the treasures held by the five *zang*.
>
> *Suwen*, Chapter 23

> The Heart stores the Spirits, the Lung stores the Breaths, the Liver stores the Blood, the Spleen stores the Flesh *rou* 肉 , and the Kidneys store the Will. Thus is the body formed.
>
> *Suwen*, Chapter 62

Clearly we see two parallel explanations. Chapter 23 is looking at the way the higher life of man is expressed. Here the *Po*, the *Hun*, and the Intent *yi* fall into line between the Heart and the Kidneys. On the other hand, Chapter 62 observes the constitution of the body as a way by which the *Hun* and the *Po* (also placed between the Heart and the Kidneys) express their own life. Several things could be said, especially regarding a certain duality of the role of the Heart (which remains always the residence of the Spirits) and the Kidneys (which thesaurize all the celestial and earthly aspects of Will). We will not elaborate this point here. We prefer to draw attention to the normal substitution of Blood for the *Hun*, and Breaths for the *Po*, when those explaining are concerned more with the physical functioning of corporeal life than with the higher level of the being.

When something takes charge of the beings we speak of the Heart . (line 25)

In chapter 8 of the *Suwen*, Qi Bo's task is to present life methodically as it functions in an organized being. Twelve functions or "charges" work in concert. In the lead because of its dignity, and also in the center because of its position as ruler, is the Heart.

The heart has the charge of being Sovereign and master;
the shining radiance of the Spirits comes forth from it.

The presentation in Chapter 8 of the *Lingshu* has the same quality. Sober and powerfully articulated, the language serves an even broader perspective. One is present at the constitution of the human "me," from the moment that virtue pours forth from Heaven. This virtue is transformed, and the term for the transformation is knowing-how. The individuals that we are are so many "hearts" where the impulse of Heaven/Earth meet. Man is the heart of the Universe, and his "empty" heart takes responsibility for the movement of beings. We risk proposing a formula that may seem obscure:

The Heart of Man is the Heart of the Universe.

In every man, the heart takes the function of the Overlord of the State. Happiness or unhappiness, illness or health, longevity or premature death all depend on the heart. A wounded body evokes the image of an oppressed, tyrannized people, detesting and cursing its prince. The heart must be healthy to fulfill what is obvious to the Chinese, and yet what is a contradiction for other minds: that the heart can hold, take the burden of, all beings, while itself remaining absolutely empty. For the heart, the fullness of life is emptiness. The individual life is centered by the heart which creates a composition of harmonious breaths, reassembling and reuniting the constituents of a being. The heart assumes the serene authority appropriate to the sovereign who has mastery. Stable and safe in the interior, it is in a fit state to "take on the burden of all beings."

Taking on the Responsibility

The texts warn us not to overload the heart. The heart fills without knowing it. As soon as we are aware of this fullness which is always bad — perhaps mortally dangerous — we must empty our heart. Its movement of filling and encumbering itself is natural, since it is given to it "to take on the charge of other beings." We are in the world, of course, and we are here to deal with it, but life is a gushing forth whose power and clearness at the source must be protected. Our movement toward the outside is the principal danger to our own longevity, through draining contact with the beings among whom we live. Intense use of the senses is to be proscribed because it "throws the heart into turmoil." We must make haste to learn to unlearn, in order to reach non-knowing and to act only through non-action. This negation, whose effects reinforce our vitality, is obtained through what we currently call renunciation. This word "renunciation" does not mean the destruction of oneself or the negation of others, or rejection of the exterior world, but is a judicious husbanding of the relationship between the foundations of vitality and the demands of the senses with whatever perversions follow along at their heels. As the text is gradually discussed and explained, there will be plenty of time to see what this means. For now, it is sufficient to name the relationship of the heart to all beings, and to say how the heart takes on the burden. In the West we also say that the heart is made for carrying the burdens of others. The Chinese position is far more radical, more ontological: the heart is not made for taking on the burden; it is, itself, the taking on of the burden. To be and to do are identified through the vitalist perspective of Daoism. To live is nothing more than the perpetually renewed equalizing of doing and being. We have nothing else to do than to be. The life of each being is authentic only insofar as it is carried by the natural movement that gives birth to the Ten Thousand Beings that are the radiant lineage of Heaven and of Earth.

Nothing exists that is not "taken on." "To take on" is *ren* 任 . In the Wieger etymology (*Wieger* Lesson 82C) a man, shown as a simple vertical line, carries a burden formed of two balanced loads hung from the two ends of a yoke, a piece of flexible wood placed upon the shoulders. Heaven is the ultimately responsible one, the great carrier. Man is the image of Heaven. That aspect in man which "takes on the burden of all beings" is called heart.

In this system of explaining the world, the modalities of the Virtue of Heaven are laid out in an ensemble of five couples. They are called "celestial trunks" or "heavenly stems" *tian gan* 天干. The ninth and tenth trunks, which are *ren* 壬 and *gui* 癸 , deal with fecundity. Fecundity is composed of the pivot point that "takes on the burden," and also of actual conception. One immediately thinks of the liquid fire out of which life arises. This is important, but it is probably not sufficient. There is only the materiality of an uncontestable reality that is universal and too simple to be explained. In returning to the origins of beings – to Creative Heaven – our effort to see clearly must collide with the evidence of the fact that we exist. It is safer to stay with the picturesque image of bearing/carrying. All the loads of the world are suspended from the transverse pole that moves with the forward movement of the great bearer. We can complete this imagery, adding to *ren* 壬 a silhouette of a woman *nü* 女. The bearing of the burden is now oriented toward the procreation – out of the woman's body –of a new being, this burden she carries for which she is responsible. The heavenly Virtue is superactivated in her. She can no longer distinguish between the being she is and the being she carries. It is the same with the heart.

The heart is celestial virtue, perceived as the virtue that bears beings *wu* 物 . Who are the *wu*? All that is not the heart will be called *wu*, beings. Certainly the text mentions *wu* in order to distinguish between the heart and all that penetrates (and is reflected by) the heart. *Wu* is the equivalent of *wan wu* 萬物, the Ten Thousand Beings. The affairs, the range of the being, and (by the incessant movement of *hun* and *po*) the exchanges of breaths that make up the particular life carried along in the universal flood are all part of the Ten Thousand Beings. A sovereign prince, the Emperor, is first of all an ordinary citizen. Above all he takes on the burden of himself; but his vigilant and tranquil activity takes on the destiny of all that is under Heaven. He carries everything in his heart.

> When that which occupies the center, *zhong* 中 , is a perfectly regulated heart *zheng xin* 正心 , the Ten Thousand Beings *wan wu* obtain fair measure *du* 度 (no excess).
>
> *Guanzi*, Chapter 49, *Neiye*

What underlies this place of the heart is its being the dwelling place of the Spirits, making it the intermediary between the power of Heaven and the multitude sheltered by its authority. In the individual the heart is the son of Heaven, the image of Heaven, suggesting to man that he mold himself to Earth, to Heaven, and to Nature.

> The heart has the responsibility of Sovereign and master; it gathers and presides over the Spirits and their beneficent influences *shen ling* 神靈, and it places itself in a triad with Heaven and Earth; in this way it takes on the burden of the Ten Thousand Beings.
>
> *Zhang Jiebin*

The light of the Heavenly Spirits allows the heart to be the starting place of all reaction and all knowledge, to assure cohesion of conduct. Thus the importance of an "Art of the Heart" *xin shu* 心術 that functions in serenity and calm, like the clear transparence of still water mirroring the reality of beings and things. If agitation rules, everything is stirred up and nothing is clear. How can one have understanding? How can one regulate conduct and emotions?

> From the first moment of his existence, a man's heart is in a place of the most absolute calm (it is free of all desire); Heaven creates it in this state. Soon external objects act on it and produce diverse movements; these are desires that add themselves to its nature (to its original state).
>
> In the presence of external objects, man has the faculty (or the desire) to know them; when he knows them, he experiences feelings of attraction for some and feelings of revulsion for others. If he does not master these feelings, he lets himself be drawn towards external things and becomes incapable of returning within himself (and regulating the movements of his heart); he loses the good tendencies he has received from Heaven.
>
> *Liji*, Couvreur translation, II, p. 52, *Yueji*

Good government, which is the taking on of responsibilities, belongs to the heart.

> By nature man possesses blood and breaths, and a heart that allows knowledge. Grief as well as joy and elation as well as anger do not exist permanently in him; they are reactions to the incitement of objects. It is then that the Art of the Heart *xin shu* intervenes.
>
> *Liji, Yueji*

The Art of the Heart consists of making the heart a center that can receive all the incitements and yet remain in conformity with nature *xing* 性 [17] in such a way that feelings are only the essences expressed in the way the subtle breaths work. The feelings are *qing* 情 .[18]

In a calm and empty heart nothing gets thoughtlessly attached, nothing occupies the place unduly or besieges the heart, blocking and

---

[17]*Xing* is the heart and life, the proper nature of a being. See Glossary.

[18]*Qing* is the heart and the verdant hues of ascending life. The composition of the ideogram *qing*, feelings, is similar to that of the ideogram *jing*, essences; the radical changes, and the heart takes the place of the grain of rice. See Glossary.

encumbering it; but everything comes forward and is received to be weighed and assessed.

>How can a person know the Dao? By the heart.

>How can the heart know? By emptiness, the pure attention that unifies being and quietude *xu yi jing* 虛壹靜.

>The heart is never without treasure *cang* 藏 , yet it is called empty *xu* 虛.

>The heart is never not completely filled *man* 滿, yet it is called unified *yi* 壹 .[19]

>The heart is never without movement *dong* 動 , yet it is called quiet *jing* 靜 .

>Man lives and possesses knowledge *zhi* 知 ; he knows, and through knowledge possesses will *zhi* 志.

>Will is thesaurization (active and careful storing of precious treasure). However, the heart is called empty, for emptiness has nothing to do with impressions already gathered, but with what is going to be received.

>The heart is alive *sheng* 生 ,[20] and it possesses knowledge; it knows, and from knowing makes distinctions. To make distinctions is to know all parts of the whole at once.

>At rest, the heart dreams *meng* 夢 ; in calmness *yu* 俞 it behaves naturally *zi xing* 自行; when in action *shi* 使, it makes plans *mo* 謨 . For this reason the heart is never without some movement *dong* 動 ; but it is called quiet. This quietude is there because dreams do not disarrange the consciousness.

>*Xunzi*, Chapter 21, *Jiebi*

Calm and quietude, the Art of the Heart, are not the denial of the movements and reactions that make up life. On the contrary, the Art of the Heart is analysis of these movements and reactions. It is the temperance that distances anger and outbursts. It is the perpetual re-establishment of a balance made of breaths and blood, flesh and bone, feelings and thought.

The heart's grandeur is the pure and clear perception of true consciousness. Thus can the heart take on the burden of beings.

---

[19] *Yi*, a concentration of pure attention.
[20] Life.

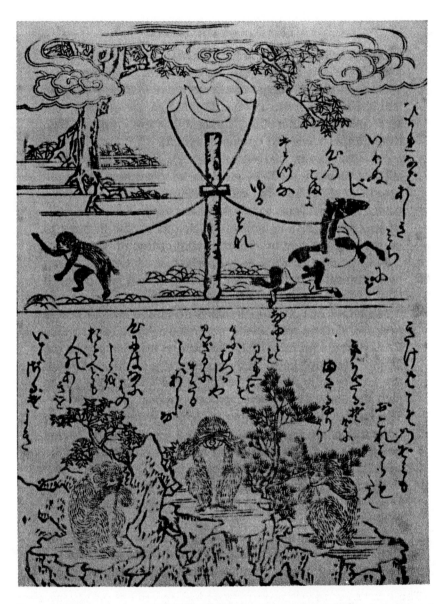

The art of the heart consists of maintaining firmly one's heart-anchor in peace and correctness, solid as a tree trunk, the pillar in the center of the picture. One must not allow oneself to be carried away by trembling passions or by the quickness of too much ardor, symbolized here by the thoroughbred horse. One must not abandon oneself to the never-assuaged desires of the senses, represented here by the three monkeys.

The Art of the Heart

The heart is the sovereign-master *zhu* 主 of the Five *Zang*. It regulates and permits the activity of the Four Members. Through it the blood and the breaths *xue qi* flow and circulate; the spaces of yes and no *shi fei* 是非 are overrun by it at a full gallop; the One Hundred Matters come and go through the doors and openings *men hu* 門戶 .

For this reason, one who, not having full possession *de* 得 of his heart, meddles at imposing norms *jing* 經 on the breaths *qi* of the Empire, can be compared to a person who, having no ears, claims to tune bells and drums, or to one who, lacking vision, says he enjoys art. Neither is able to bring to completion the role he claims to take charge of *ren* 任.

This sacred vase *shen qi* 神器 which is the Empire cannot be manipulated by one's will. He who would manipulate it fails; it escapes the one who would grasp it.

We know that Xu You attached no importance to power over the Empire and would never have consented to take Yao's position for himself. He had not set his heart *zhi* on the Empire. How do I know this? I answer: one is concerned with the Empire only from the reality of the Empire. For essentially the Empire is not separate, but is within oneself *wo* 我. The Empire is not in another individual *ren* 人 , but is in what makes me myself, *wo shen* 我身 , and only by having possession of myself *de* 得, can I bring the community of the Ten Thousand Beings to perfection.

The serious practitioner of the Art of the Heart *xin shu* keeps lust and desires at a distance, and also attractions and revulsions.

From this we see that the bringing up of excessive joy *xi* 喜[21] and anger *nu* 怒, or of deep joy *le* 樂 and bitterness *ku* 苦, are for the Ten Thousand Beings primitive communion *xuan tong* 玄同 that must be neither affirmed nor denied, but must move through the transformations *hua*, nourish and reach the mystical brightness, living a life that looks like death.

Huainanzi, Chapter 1

---

[21] Elation, exhilaration.

The vital thrust is directed by the heart with sovereign authority. The heart expands in its surroundings, which we call the body, and which classical tradition calls the Four Members. The five *zang* are the marvelous engine of the organic reconstruction of life under the guidance of the five authorities.[22] The symbiosis of the blood and breaths always confers, by authority of the heart, a vivifying power to the organic ensemble. We could also say that cosmic life flows out and circulates in us under the connecting and contrasting modalities of the blood and the breaths.

It would seem ridiculous to an educated Chinese not to include in the act of animation whatever it is that gives dignity to the act and underlies its power. We must understand that every man is fully alive only through this inner structure of the heart, intelligent and willing, capable of determinations and decisions. These decisions are taken under the influence of likes and dislikes (attractions and revulsions), and cause us to go through the space of life fully in every sense, and at a lively pace.

This is a unified and vast movement, like a destiny dividing itself into days, and according to the vicissitudes of the daily management of the One Hundred Matters. We enter and exit this movement by doors and openings which remind us that an organic basis is always required for the most moral of activities.

The heart is surely this Sovereign, surrounded by its court. Normally withdrawn to the interior, it communicates with the exterior without itself being disturbed, even when the effect it creates − the animation of the Empire − is felt everywhere. Via the sense organs the heart (or in other words, the interior) may communicate with the exterior and with the business of the world. This communication is a movement of ceaseless goings and comings.

When the Heart applies itself, we speak of Intent. *(line 26)*

An examination follows of the ideograms representing "applies itself" and "intent."

"To apply oneself" *yi* 憶 is formed by the ideogram for "intent" *yi* 意, to which is added − for the second time − the radical for heart 心. This radical for the heart already appears in the ideogram for intent *yi*, written at the bottom of the ideogram.

---

[22] *Shen*/Heart, *Hun*/Liver, *Po*/Lung, Intent/Spleen, and Will (or Essences)/Kidneys.

Yi 憶. has the active meaning of thought that arises, that recollects the self, that recalls one's spirit. From this comes the idea of a kind of application of the spirit that takes into account what comes to itself, what presents itself.

Yi 意. has the meaning of intent, idea, thought, opinion, meaning, intention, taste, and tendency. In current language the ideogram is completed by another ideogram, in order to better establish the aspect one wants to draw out from the series of possible meanings.

Let us analyze and study the ideogram *yi* 意, intent. It is composed of the heart 心 placed beneath the musical note *yin* 音 , which is a celestial vibration that Heaven bestows on a breath produced by a being. The heart recognizes if the vibration coming to it is true, that is, if its nature is such that the heart can compose with it. The heart holds the position of composer and orchestra conductor, and also choir master. It recognizes compatibility, the primary requirement for anything's taking form.

The heart, aware of itself, accepts or rejects what is being presented to it. Is the thing presented to the heart true, and is it the right tone? The heart applies itself to whatever comes to it, in order to identify, recognize, and either make it its own or reject it.

There is nothing fixed in "intent," no formalized "firm intent". Intent grows out of the formulation that follows the proposition.[23] It will become fixed or determined in a later stage.

Because it is vacant and calm, the empty and serene heart receives all the thoughts that germinate there like mushrooms. It takes care not to be affected by them; it sorts out the rye grass seed and only lets those grow that will be to its advantage. Supported by the heart, the germ of processes of conscience, of knowledge, and of action can develop.

> Are there any unprofitable affairs? Those from which
>   the heart does not profit.
> Is there a place of no peace? When the heart is not at
>   peace.
> In the center of the heart, there is another heart.
> Intent *yi* precedes declaration *yan* 言
> After intent comes form *xing* 形
> After form comes thought *si* 思.
> After thought comes knowledge *zhi* 知.

---

[23] The proposition stated in line 26.

> In every case where the heart is encumbered by
> formalized knowledge, life is lost *shi sheng* 失生
> *Guanzi*, Chapter 37, *Xinshu, The Art of the Heart*

The "heart within the heart" is the emptiness of the heart, the innermost of the inner. Even the syntactic construction may indicate an empty space that is fathomless.

Let us accumulate and store the essences in the interior and let us constitute an inexhaustible source for the Spirits of life. Through free communication, this lively wellspring helps the heart guarantee its effective charge over beings. It brings about harmony between the parts, detecting all dissonance, avoiding the cacophony engendered by offence to the natural (heavenly) dispositions constituting the nature of each being.

This recognition by the heart brings on the appearance of what we call "Intent" *yi*. Intent is a focal point, a concentration affected by the heart. This concentration allows form to occur; that which was presented to the heart is now represented by the outlines of a form: word, discussion, acts, work, conduct.

The heart is behind every act of knowledge *zhi*, but in the way that the Sovereign and the master are behind the multiple work of administration and the countless tasks of the people.

The conformity of Intent to the heart is repeated and ceaseless:

> Empty the heart and balance the intent, and you will enjoy natural conduct.
> *Guanzi*, Chapter 55

> With unity and will concentrated in the heart, ears and eyes protected from perverse infiltrations, what is faraway seems near.
> *Guanzi*, Chapter 49, *Neiye*

When Intent becomes permanent, we speak of Will. (line 27)

Through Will the heart chooses, in the compost of memory and of life lived, to present something that is fixed and determined. Determination proceeds from this. The power of the kidneys is now going to be added to the power of the spleen, the latter of which expresses itself well through Intent: formalization, recollection, richness of terrain. The kidneys are the stable foundation, the possibility of firmly establishing an idea, and of strongly stabilizing a new presentation.

The character *cun* 存 indicates this dwelling within a being that keeps alive and maintains dispositions or intentions that have not yet been anchored.

The union of Intent *yi* 意 and Will *zhi* 志 is found in the everyday expressions *zhi yi* or *yi zhi*. They accent the fact that the two are joined, bringing to whatever is being formed strength of germination and structural support and the internal tension that will animate it. This joining echoes that of Anterior Heaven and Posterior Heaven, of which kidneys and spleen are the representatives; there we have the complementarity of these two powers to express what has not yet appeared, but which will underlie the advent of thought.

Will *zhi* is a movement initiated in the heart, but nothing appears, nothing comes out of the heart; the act has not yet begun; the Will is the antecedent of all precise feeling, of all constructed thought.

In this sense, the Will anchors the feelings, and the feelings are the expression of the movement appropriate to each of the five *zang*: each one regulates itself in relation to the others and participates in the regulation of the others. By the generic name of *wu zhi* 五志 we designate the Five Wills, the ensemble formed by the feelings of anger (impetus, vehemence), elation (joyous excitation), thought (preoccupation), chagrin (depletion), and fear. In Chapter 5 of the *Suwen* they are the expression — at the level of feelings — of the aspect of life that forms and maintains the *zang*; the liver, heart, spleen, lung, and kidneys.

In Chapter 8 of the *Lingshu* the emotions are the focus of the second part, where their pathological aspect is considered. When the emotions are in balance, nothing has affect for long; one does not remain in any one emotion.

Here, the Will has its place in the process that leads the mystery of life to efficacious and controlled conduct. The vital tension announces and precedes sudden appearances. Will applies itself to life in the first instance. It is the will-to-life. It then achieves all that life, through the heart, recognizes as true, acceptable, and favorable.

One's orientation, already apparent in Intent, is affirmed and becomes directive. But we must guard against intellectualizing the Will. Its beginnings are before thought, before reflection, before meditation. However, there is nothing thoughtless about it. It is impulse, the natural and vital impulse in me, the injection of the vital life forces. It comes from the guts and the lower belly but resonates perfectly with the Intent and with the Heart.

When the persevering will changes, we speak of Thought. (line 28)

The commentators have clearly established the meaning of this:

> That will perseveres but changes, means that the ensemble formed by intent and will *yi zhi*, though itself a fixed thing, turns the data over and over, calculating, computing, and measuring – this is thought.
>
> *Zhang Jiebin*

> The concentrated and persevering will changes and re-volves, seeking different positions. This is thought.
>
> *Taisu*

We seek all possible mutations and alterations, but do so without drifting. Our anchorage, orientation, direction and purpose, once cho-sen, remain unquestioned. We compute and calculate for efficiency, but we do so on stable and sure foundations. We inspect the many facets of a new project, inspiration, or idea, but we must not toy with it. The inability to stay with an idea is a pathological symptom, as is the inability ever to change anything when a new era is heralded or when circumstances have changed.

The Chinese find nourishment in the *Book of Changes* (*Yijing*). True thought exists only in the appreciation of circumstances and in adap-tation to the time and circumstances. What might have been called opportunism is only a vitalistic realism.

To assure the noblest function of the human being, which is thought, the following are necessary: the full presence of the Spirits and the full powers of the subtlest essences, all together in the highest extremity of the individual, which is the brain and the head, with the subtle sense organs.

Thought knows no hesitation but dwells on reflection. One returns to the issue, perceives better the questions that arise, but does not return to reconsider the principle, for one knows what he wants and where he is headed before knowing the details.

The beginning of the *Book of History* (*Annals, Shujing*) attributes four great virtues to the mythic Emperor Yao. Thought *si* is one of them:

> (Yao) was constantly attentive to fulfilling his duty *qin* 欽 ;[24]
> he was very perspicacious *ming* 明 ,[25] of high virtue *wen* 文 and rare prudence *si* 思, all naturally and effortlessly.
>
> *Shujing, The Canon of Yao*, Couvreur translation, p.1

A commentator, also translated by Couvreur, explains these last two virtues:

> *Wen*: his thoughts and his sentiments were all admirably arranged and formed like a magnificent fabric.
>
> *Si*: he combined his plans with profound wisdom.
>
> These four virtues, innate in him, had their root in his very nature. They were not the fruit of great effort, and he practiced them with ever-growing ease.

Another commentary simply says:

> When the Way and the Virtue *dao de* 道德 are perfectly pure and ready to be effective, we speak of thought *si*.

When Thought extends itself powerfully and far, we speak of Reflection.[26] (line 29)

> When Thought, which was changing and searching, reverses and turns toward the future (forges ahead), then this is Reflection.
>
> *Taisu*

That is theoretical perfection. Other commentaries are wary of the dangers of "weighing anchor" at that level:

> If one thinks too deeply and goes too far into the distance, crippling doubts will inevitably appear.
>
> *Zhang Jiebin*

When thoughtfulness has been far and deep and has branched broadly, if the rooting remains solid and firmly attached in the heart, thought can develop into projects.

---

[24] Assiduous and vigilant.
[25] Of penetrating intelligent.
[26] Meditation, contemplation.

Lü 慮 , reflection, belongs to the liver, as *si*, thought, belongs to the spleen. Simple thought reflects upon elements already experienced. Lessons are drawn from the experience; we meditate, and more precisely, we cogitate. We draw from the compost of the already-seen, the already-lived, the yield of learned and assimilated experiences. The spleen has the role of digesting, assimilating, and transporting all the way to the extremities.

Lü: we project towards the future to fulfill what has not yet been. In Chapter 8 of the *Suwen* (cf *The Secret Treatise of the Spiritual Orchid*), the liver fulfilling its function of being the Commanding General and Commander of the Armies, analyzes the circumstances and conceives its plans *mou lü* 謀慮 as a result. The same ideogram *lü* is used to designate the conception of plans. The liver has a long reach with its impetuous energy. It forges ahead. Nothing can go so far, in so brief a time, as vision.

In the same way that Liver/Wood assists in the expansion of Spleen/Earth for all circulations to be carried out well and all functions accomplished, thought is also completed by reflection, which carries thought far and simultaneously augments its power.

Lü does not know unstructured projects, ingenious and brilliant ideas that pass through the brain without remaining there; *lü* is the inverse — the conception of a plan, the determining of an attitude, of conduct, when the Heart, Intent, Will, and Thought, are all in their place and remain there.

Lü is both broad meditation and intense calculation on precise objectives. It is activity of the spirit that is firmly anchored and at the same time overflowing with vitality. Meditation is the exemplary aspect of the power that is life; it can never drift, nor break with Will, Thought, Heart, and Intent. Meditation abhors fantasy and requires the heart to fast.

Deep meditation prepares, in absolute silence, the springing forth of plans, calculated to the finest detail, ready to be fulfilled immediately. These are the two sides of thought. Tigers and men — men often being seated on a tiger skin to meditate — share the power of Earth proportionately to their nature. But men leap farther than tigers when they allow themselves to be guided by the Virtue of Heaven.

When Reflection can have all beings at its disposal, we speak of Knowing-How. (line 30)

Zhi 智 (knowing, knowing-how) is the first ideogram since the appearance of the Heart that does not have the radical for the heart 心, but that for the sun 日. Through a multiplicity of stages the radiance of the Spirits gives light to life and creates an enlightened consciousness, a unified and just word, knowledge, and efficiency.

The spirits are unchangeable and inexhaustible: either they are there, or they leave us. The essences are exhaustible. Knowing-how is the good conduct of life. It is most often found in relation to the kidneys or the spleen, which are precisely the two *zang* most concerned with the essences — the kidneys for their maintenance, and the spleen for the source of their renewal.

There is wise caution and prudence in *zhi*. In modern Chinese the expression *zhi lü* 智慮 means prudent doubt. The rapport between the two notions is clarified by the commentator Zhang Jiebin:

> When uncertainty and reflection appear, one moves toward the better of them, and that is knowing-how.

Beaming another light on the ideogram *lü*, we understand that it assembles the meanings of reflection, doubt, uncertainty, and meditation, and we understand how, through reflection, one can have all the beings at one's disposal *chu* 庶.

The *Shiming* explains *lü*, reflection, by using the homophone, *lü* 旅. This *lü* means to travel, to be away from one's home; it also means a military formation, a brigade. One lays things out in order, as one arranges things according to protocol. This *lü* is also the fifty-sixth hexagram of the *Book of Changes (Yijing)*, and it is called The Wanderer, defined thus:

> When the beings are no longer in their appropriate place, they diligently seek support. Perseverance furthers.

This clarifies *lü*, reflection, and its capacity to arrange all beings. If reflection is only a wandering of mind and thought, nothing can be ordered or arranged, and nothing can take its relative place and prepare for action. This is not appropriate reflection. It is loss of identity, of the established conscience, of one's naturally happy frame of mind, and of what is compatible with it. Beings, things, ideas and thoughts have lost their natural place. Reflection, which should put them in order, is wandering.

If, on the contrary, *lü* is a time of reflection upon the action to take, everything finds its appropriate order, and anxiety is replaced by assurance. There is a putting into form, which is a putting of everything and everyone into its adequate form. Each of the innumerable ideas, thoughts, circumstances, and stimuli finds its own place which is its natural locus, its rung in the hierarchy.

When certitude is lacking for arranging beings and circumstances, the reflection that brings order is prudent uncertainty. It is the anxiety experienced when the heart gets thrown off track, when it does not have enough power to make *lü* a real reflection, and when, in the same manner, it lacks power so that thought *si* is only a repetitious turning over and over of the same thing. Power (that reaches forcefully and far) defines reflection; it is through this power that reflection is capable of arranging beings in a way that allows knowing-how to appear. Without it, everything is reduced to a deep hindering of body and spirit:

> The man whose reflection *lü* does not unfurl powerfully
> *wu yuan* 無遠 is very close to exhaustion *you* 憂.
> *Analects of Confucius, Lunyu*, 7.15.11

Let us now give to Qi Bo's last statement a unifying commentary, destined to give value to the passage from "Thought," through the movement of "Reflection," to "Knowing-how." Then we shall examine each ideogram in the light of traditional etymologies, to better grasp the teaching called up again by Qi Bo.

The work of the whole of life is to accomplish longevity. To attain that, one must know how to do it. Each being accomplishes the number of his days, and the internal Sovereign rules peaceably, governing the health of the Empire to the degree that his ability to maintain existence proceeds from "Knowing-how" within him and around him. The "knowing" must go as far as the "how-to-do." Only the knowing appearing in the doing translates realistically the breadth of thought and the power of reflection.

The civilization constructed brilliantly by the Chinese demonstrates the marvelously realistic gift of the peasants, as well as of the royal court, to direct the life of the nation intelligently. This power of the arts and techniques, of meditation on politics and the rites belonging to them, is an astonishing aptitude for mastering the free flight of thought by the constraining power of reflection, and it leads thought to the satisfactory disposal of everything.

With the resources of the virtue of Heaven by which we are invested, lifted up, and organized, each of us is solicited to respond (by attentive treatments and exact conduct) to expected situations that press in from every side. But the ultimate goal of life is not to know about the behavior of beings, aspects of business, or bargains down to the smallest hair-splitting detail. We must act at the opportune moment. We say "beings" or "things" indifferently, in order to render the indefinite sense of *wu* 物. All that remains of Thought, when it becomes Reflection, is that it must be translated into action.

To embrace the totality of the work of arranging the whole universe, Qi Bo uses the expression *chu wu* 處物 : everything arranged and everything used. To dispose, to arrange, comprises all the degrees of passage into action. One can "accompany" the natural movement; one can "restore" the natural movement; one may be tempted to substitute oneself for the natural movement. We arrange flowers in a vase, guests around a table, a nest for a pair of birds. But one also arranges a daughter for her marriage, and arranges the whole of life and death of vassals and functionaries. In all cases, we speak of "knowing how to do." We arrange everything after "reflection," mature consideration, and deep speculation. But is not this "knowing-how" too external?

Reflection originates in thought. Perhaps we can compare thought to the bird Peng (*Zhuangzi*, Chapter 1, cf. *Le Vol Inutile*). Peng's life, his flight, and his "thought" all emanate from the depths of the mass of waters located in the North. They then rise powerfully to the heights, to direct themselves unfailingly toward the luminous abyss of the massed breaths located in the South. Peng flies forward with his back to the blue sky, and below him he sees the limitless landscape made up of all beings.

For another illustration, still in the magnificent style of a Chinese Gustave Doré, we turn to Chapter 17 of *Zhuangzi*. The image is no longer a bird's flight across the majestic sweep of Heaven, but the infinite expanse of the waters, the greatest of all the seas — the Ocean. Here is the grandiose panorama that reduces to nothing the pretensions of those who, having seen the small part, think they know the whole. This is the lesson of things that, showing us the narrowness of our ordinary knowledge, help us attain a true knowledge according to the Way. From this knowledge according to the Way one can derive knowing-how, through reflection:

> It was the time of the autumn flood. One hundred rivers
> were emptying their waters into the Huanghe (Yellow River),
> whose bed was so widened that one could not distinguish

between a cow or horse on the opposite bank. This sight brought joy to the Genie of the River who was elated, thinking there was nothing in the world better than his domain. Marching East following the flood, he went as far as the North sea. Gazing to the East he could not see the end of the waters. Then the Genie of the River began looking all about him to find Ruo (the Genie of the Sea) in the immensity, and he said to him with a sigh: "The adage, 'he has been instructed by the Way one hundred times, yet still he prefers himself to any other,' applies to me. I have heard it said that the teaching of Confucius was not worth much, nor the rigorous virtue of Bo Yi, and I did not believe it. But now that I have seen your unfathomable depths I have done well to come to your school; otherwise the masters of the great teachings would have ended up laughing at me."

Ruo of the North Sea answered him: "Yes, the frog that lives at the bottom of the well has no way to speak of the sea; it remains stuck in its hole. The mayfly of summer has no way to speak of ice; it is confined by its season. A scholar caught in the net of his own mind has no way to speak of the Way; he remains imprisoned by his education. Having left your narrow bed, you have seen the vast sea, and you are aware of your own smallness. You are now capable of speaking of the Great Principle of beings."

This story helps us understand, in seeing the Ocean, how immense is the Way. The change in our willing-to-know mind will be achieved through the direct confrontation with the Virtue of the Way, evoked by the Genie of the Sea. His very name, Ruo (literally meaning "who resembles") says that one perceives more than one knows or is aware of.

The spectacle of the autumn floods and the explanations of Ruo, Genie of the Sea, are a "reflection" upon knowledge and its limits. Perhaps we now understand better what is meant by "reflection." It is not enough to "think;" we must master the uncertainty that is endemic to "thought." We are led naturally, without leaving the watery domain, to learn a lesson of "knowing-how." It is a swimming lesson. We are going to learn to swim in the current. The master swimmer enters the scene:

Confucius was contemplating the countryside at Lü Liang. Plunging from thirty times a man's height, the cataract poured in a foaming torrent for 40 *li*;[27] neither tortoise nor crocodile,

---

[27] One *li* equals 1/3 mile.

nor even fish could swim in the current. Suddenly he (Confucius) saw a man swimming there. Taking him for a despondent person who had decided to drown himself, he told his disciples to go along the bank and pull him from the water. Several hundred steps farther on, the man left the water, untied his hair, and began walking along the river's edge singing. Confucius, coming up behind him, said: "I thought you were a ghost, but looking more closely, I see that you are a man. Will you tell me your secret for moving in the water?" "I have no secret," replied the man. "I began swimming with effort; when I was grown it became more natural, until I made it part of my nature. I dive in and I become one body with the water. I go with the eddies. I follow the motion of the water, not my own will. That is how I move in the water." Confucius repeated: "What do you mean: 'I began to swim with effort; when I grew up it became more natural until it became part of my nature?'" He answered: "I was born on firm ground, and therefore felt very safe on firm ground. I grew up in the water, and so felt very safe with the nature of water; but (now) I do not even know why I do what I do. It is my lot."

Zhuangzi, Chapter 19

For further discussion of the thirteen preceding ideas, see the Appendix.

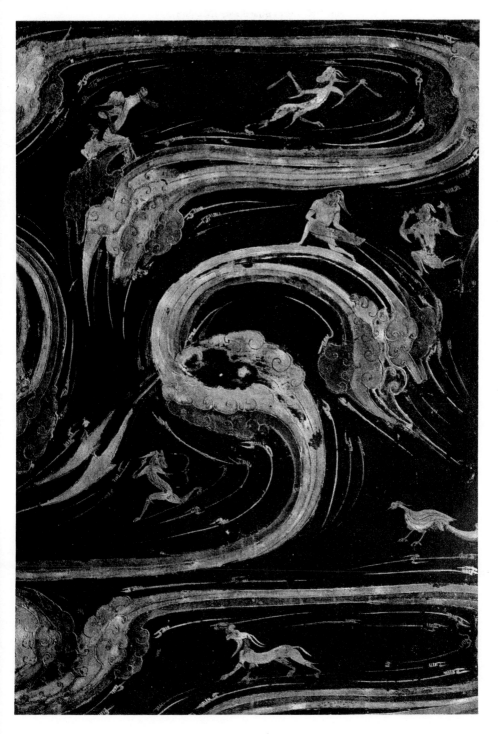

Spirits (Shen)

Translation of Characters 187 - 226, Lines 31-39

Thus, Knowing-How is the maintenance of life.
Do not fail to observe the Four Seasons
And to adapt to heat and cold,
To Harmonize elation and anger
And to be calm in activity as in rest,   35
To regulate the *yin/yang*
And to balance the hard and the soft.

In this way, having deflected the perverse energies,
There will be long life and everlasting vision.

Characters 187 to 226

故智者之養生也
gu zhi zhe zhi yang sheng ye

必順四時而適寒暑
bi shun si shi er shi han shu

和喜怒而安居處
he xi nu er an ju chu

節陰陽而調剛柔
jie yin yang er tiao gang rou

如是則僻邪不至
ru shi ze bi xie bu zhi

長生久視
chang sheng jiu shi

Thus, Knowing-How is the maintenance of life. *(line 31)*

> The effects produced indefinitely by the Spirits belong to knowing-how; and this is why knowing-how maintains life.
>
> *Taisu*

Knowing-how is knowing how to maintain one's life, to be acquainted with its rules, to respect them and avoid waste and loss. It is to hold oneself — internally and externally — in harmony with all that exists.

> The Spirits are the inexhaustible reservoir of knowing-how; when this inexhaustible reservoir is clear and pure, knowing-how shines forth. Knowing-how is the storehouse of the heart. Through perfect knowing-how, the heart is in balance.
>
> *Huainanzi*, Chapter 2

Knowing-how is a correct practice governed by the Spirits. We conform to the life of Heaven/Earth to avoid premature decline. The third chapter of *Zhuangzi* starts with the famous anecdote of Prince Liang's butcher, who is questioned by the prince on the art of maintaining the vital principle. The title of this chapter is *yang sheng zhu* 養生主 , "Principles for the Maintenance of Life."

The expression *yang sheng* 養生 , maintenance of life, is also found in Chapter 8 of the *Suwen*:

> If the sovereign (who is also the heart) is radiant (with Virtue), inferiors will be peaceable; in that way the maintenance of life will procure longevity. . . .
>
> But, if the sovereign is not radiant (with Virtue), the twelve charges (the organs) will be endangered . . . so that maintenance of life will founder in catastrophe.

The very beginning of the *Suwen* (cf. *The Way of Heaven*)[28] is an exhortation to maintain one's life well. Appropriate conduct follows the directives of the heart, and knowing-how emanates from that. Knowing-how details the things that adapt an individual perfectly to his human status between Heaven and Earth. Everything passes through the confluence of the breaths of the seasons and the passions. Everything marries a structure of bone and flesh, where emptiness and fullness alternate.

---

[28] Claude Larre, author, and Peter Firebrace, translator, *The Way of Heaven* (Cambridge: Monkey Press, 1993)

The six modes of maintaining the vital principle propose knowing-how organically; it is symbolically laid out in two-times-three propositions.

In the sequence of the thirteen propositions (lines 17 through 30, characters 84 to 186), maintenance of the vital principle holds the highest place. It is the permanent reconstitution, the tireless re-composition of the free circulations of what makes life. The heavenly Virtue flows permanently in me and the Breaths distribute it, just as Water and Fire animate the space between Heaven and Earth.

Maintenance of life *yang sheng* is inclusive in relation to other expressions led by *yang* 養 [29] in the Taoist and alchemical vocabulary:

yang qi 養氣 : to execute respiratory movements (to nourish by the particular conduct of the breaths of respiration).

yang jing 養精 : to nourish the essences.

yang shen 養神 : to nourish the spirit, the Spirits.

yang jing shen 養精神 : to nourish the essences/Spirits.

yang xing 養形 : to nourish the body.

yang xing 養性 : to nourish the vital principle, in the sense of nourishing one's own nature.

yang shen 養身 : to take care of one's health, of one's person.

yang zhen 養真 : to nourish one's authenticity, cultivate one's innate qualities.

In his essays on Taoism[30] Maspéro shows the diverse levels of these techniques for vital maintenance. He begins with a quotation from the beginning of Chapter 19 of *Zhuangzi*:

> I pity those people in the world who think that (the procedures for) "Nourishing the Body" *yang xing* 養形 are sufficient to give eternal life; in reality "Nourishing the Body" does not suffice to make life last, so how could it be sufficient for worldly people (to obtain that result)? And even though that is not sufficient for them (in order to obtain Eternal Life), they cannot do otherwise, and they cannot avoid it. Ah! those who wish

---

[29] To maintain, to nourish.

[30] Henri Maspéro, "*Essai sur le Taoïsme aux premiers siècles de l'ère chrétienne*" in *Le Taoïsme et les religions chinoises* (Paris: NRF, Gallimard, 1971).

to avoid taking care of their bodies might as well let go of the world! He who has abandoned the world has no fetters; he who is without fetters is comfortable; he who is comfortable acquires a new life; he who has a new life is near (the goal). Why is it enough to let go of the affairs (of the world)? Why is it enough to give up life? (Because) when one lets go of the affairs (of the world), the body does not tire; when one gives up life, the essence is not exhausted. Ah! when the body is complete and the essence renewed, one is One with Heaven.

And Maspéro explains:

In summation, in contrast to the method consisting of "Nourishing the Body" yang xing, or "Nourishing Life" yang sheng 養生 through physical procedures, Zhuangzi proposes a less material method, which —without excluding the former as, after all, the body must last in order to live — nevertheless rejects the physical elements on the second level, and places ahead of those a whole series of spiritual practices, particularly the work of spiritual concentration. It is through spiritual procedures, concentration, ecstasy, and the mystical union with the Dao that the Adept achieves immortality.

A little farther on in Chapter 19 of *Zhuangzi*, another quotation clarifies the Daoist position by means of a fable:

Those who understand how to maintain life yang sheng are like shepherds; when one of their sheep lags behind, they flog it to make it join the flock.
"What does that mean?" asked Duke Wei.
"This," said Tian Kaizhi. "In the kingdom of Lu, a certain Shan Bao spent his life in the mountains, drinking only water, having no contact with others. Thanks to this regimen, at the age of seventy he was still as fresh as a baby. Unfortunately, he was killed and eaten by a hungry tiger.
"There was a certain Zhang Yi [a physician]. Rich and poor people alike discussed his consultations. At the age of forty he died of an internal fever, *nei re* 内熱.
"Shan Bao maintained his interior being *yang qi nei* 養其内 but allowed his exterior being to be devoured *shi qi wai* 食其外. Zhang Yi maintained his exterior being *yang*

qi wai 養其外 but let his internal being be destroyed by disease *bing gong qi nei* 病攻其內 These two masters were wrong not to flog their lagging sheep."

Do not fail to observe the Four Seasons
And to adapt to heat and cold, *(lines 32, 33)*

The four seasons, as the alternation of *yin* and *yang*, are "the end and beginning of the Ten Thousand Beings, the rooting of death and life" (*Suwen*, Chapter 2). The seasons present simultaneously the necessity and the model for alternation and for *yin/yang* co-penetration; they show, by the manner in which earth and nature behave, how to react to cold or to heat, and how to conduct oneself when the forces of life leap forth with vigor, or when harshness arrives. This is the entire subject of Chapter 2 of the *Suwen* and is a theme that is repeated ceaselessly.

Health, vitality, and longevity are obtained by one who does not swim against the current, but who flows along in the current that life manifests around oneself in this moment, in this time. To know how to take all the storms and to resist a tenacious and penetrating humidity is a safeguard without parallel. Strengths are economized, the peaceful Spirits maintain their control, everything continues to circulate and to regenerate itself without attack on the subtle mechanism of life.

This is what it is to "observe," *shun* 順 , to follow the natural current (being able to recognize how it is at present, and knowing the paths to take to conform to it).

The four seasons are the rhythm that Heaven imprints upon the unfolding of the breaths; heat and cold are the principal effects felt on Earth and in man. The four seasons are what they are, heavenly and natural. We will take them as they come; we will recognize them and feel the balance that each represents; we will prolong in ourselves, for ourselves, what they show of themselves.

Man, capable of transformation in the Middle Void (the median space between Heaven and Earth), adapts to cold and to heat in such a way that he is not affected excessively by the effects of extreme cold or extreme heat, because he is somehow pre-adapted. Thus the sweet warmth of life is conserved without alteration or accident.

Through this adaptation that is perpetual change and mutation, the Sage – or the man who is careful of his health – takes his place in the Universal Order, which alone guarantees constancy and perenniality.

> Ah! the virtue of the Mystery, how deep it goes, how far it goes,
> How it restores beings and finally lines them up in the Universal Order *da shun* 大順.
>
> *Laozi*, Chapter 65

The *Book of Rites* (*Liji*) resonates with the same exhortation to observe the Universal Order:

> When the four members are in their normal state, and the dermis and epidermis are full, the body is in a good state. (In the same way) when father and son love each other truly . . . when the high ministers observe the laws . . . when the prince and his subjects discharge their mutual duties, the government is in a good state. When the Son of Heaven takes virtue for his carriage and music for his coachman . . . and all subjects watch over each other, being on good terms with each other, the whole Empire is in a good state. This is called the great conformity (to natural law) *da shun* 大順.
>
> When this great conformity *da shun* exists, the living are maintained everywhere *yang shen* 養生 , the dead are buried, and the spirits *gui shen* 鬼神 honored. Great things, despite their number, are accomplished without hindrance; they march abreast without the least error. The smallest things are carried out without any negligence, and there is space between the larger things. Those following each other do not touch. They move along without colliding. This is the highest degree of conformity (to natural law) *shun*.
>
> He who well understands *ming* 明 this conformity *shun* can save himself from all harm in the midst of peril.
>
> *Liji*, VII, 4, S. Couvreur Translation, I, pp. 533,534

From the moment the harmony *he* 和 of the passions, and the heart's joy *le* 樂 are upset, one is soon invaded by desires of self-interest and by concealment. The moment that maintenance ceases to be composed and respectful, laziness and carelessness slip into the heart.

Thus music *yue* 樂 acts upon man's interior *nei* 內 , and ceremonies *li* 禮 upon his exterior *wai* 外 . The goal of music is harmony *he*; the goal of ceremonies is conformity *shun* with the order of nature. When a prince's passions are in harmony *nei he* 內和 and his exterior conforms with the laws of Nature *wai shun* 外順 , the people see the look on his face, upon his countenance, and do not resist him. . . .

Liji, XXI, 1. S. Couvreur translation, II, pp. 297-298

To Harmonize elation and anger
And to be calm in rest as in activity, *(lines 34, 35)*

We would have liked to offer the reader a pleasanter translation. We have chosen a laborious expression in the hope of preserving, aside from general meaning, the articulation of each element of the original Chinese text.

Elation *xi* 喜 is not simply the *feeling* of joyous excitement that we all know at certain moments in a day, in a season, or in life. It is an *acceleration* of the vital flux which is felt at all the stages of the being and which, in the world of emotions, is a lively joy.

One should beware of this lively joy. Most men search for lively joy because they are happy with the vibration that is propagated in their souls. A Sage feels the emotion, but does not let himself be carried away. He is neither more, nor less, natural in these states of excitement, but he is attentive to them. We envy this admirable mastery of the self, although there is also something to be said against excessive surveillance of the movements of the heart.

Anger, *nu* 怒 , is not really anger; it is a violence and a vehemence. It is the opposite of lively joy, though related to the latter by its equally excessive aspect. The things that have been said about elation *xi* can also be said about anger: one should beware of this anger. Many allow themselves to be unconsciously carried away by vehemence and fury whether it is against themselves, against others, or against the "order of the world," and whether it is expressed violently or held inside with great effort.

Elation and anger must be harmonized *he* 和 . This does not so much mean that elation must be balanced by anger, or the reverse. What must be harmonized is the productive flood of joy which, reversed, is the same flood — anger.

We must also remember that joy and anger are two emotions nominally expressed here, but they stand for the totality of the emotions and passions. Similarly, heat and cold are most often named to stand for all the nuances of meteorology.

Finally, since we shall have known how to harmonize joy and anger at the wellspring of emotions and feelings, our work of intervention in the world of beings will be marked by the sign of tranquillity. Tranquil rest is not laxity; tranquil work leaves busyness behind.

Interior equilibrium translates as conduct that is constant and calm; the peace of the Spirits is reflected in all of one's attitudes.

The Four Seasons that give rhythm to our external weather imply an active harmonization, an internal adaptation to heat and cold, whereas the emotions which are born in a man's heart manifest their balance in external attitudes. It is not simply a matter of being active in opportune seasons and resting during times of scorching heat or great cold, but above all to firmly maintain the stability of one's line of conduct, through all the required adaptations and transformations. We thus conform (*shun*) to the exterior, and we harmonize (*he*) the interior.

It is not a matter of just abstaining from one's passions (elation, anger), commonly considered harmful and disturbing. It is, more subtly, a question of maintaining in temperance and sincerity throughout one's entire life, the profound accord between one's human nature and the good sense shown by the rationality of the Spirits. One must be active and offer the fruits of one's vitality, but not "deliver" oneself totally, tied hands and feet, to anything, not even to what might superficially appear to be a way of perfection. Zhuangzi warns:

> The man affected by a great elation *da xi* 大喜 is perverted by the *yang*. A man affected by a great anger *da nu* 大怒 is perverted by the *yin*. The erratic rapport of *yin/yang* obstructs the perfect functioning of the Four Seasons; heat and cold *han re* 寒熱 in disharmony do not reach completion. The repercussions attack the person's body, provoking destabilization by elation *xi* and anger *nu*, which bring on inconsistencies in rest and activity *ju chu* 居處 . Thought *si* 思 and reflection *lü* 慮 no longer hold *bu zi de* 不自得 , so they stop along the way without achieving anything tangible. Then arrogance of intent and haughtiness of attitude develop beneath Heaven. . . .

He who gives himself to the pleasures of seeing is corrupted *yin* 淫 by colors; who gives himself to the pleasures of hearing is corrupted by sounds; who loves goodness *ren* 仁 [31] too much, upsets his virtue *de* 德 ; who loves justice *yi* 義 [32] too much, wars against reason; who has a passion for rituals *li* 禮 sins through meticulousness;   who is passionate about music *yue* 樂   falls into debauchery *yin* 淫 ; who has a passion for godliness *sheng* 聖 develops cleverness; who wants to know everything *zhi* 知   looks for the small. He who keeps himself peacefully *an* 安 within the limits of his nature and his original tendencies *xing ming zhi qing* 性命之情 may or may not indulge in these eight kinds of activity. But when one takes leave of his nature and his own tendencies, everything under Heaven is disrupted.

To regulate the yin/yang
And to balance the hard and the soft. *(lines 36, 37)*

The presence of *yin/yang* is implied in the preceding couples (heat/cold, elation/anger, rest/activity). Does it come forth again in this couple with the meaning of sexual union? So it would seem, but in a very broad fashion, with an application to the hard and the soft in corporeal life.

Hard and soft are definitive structures. They are the solid lines [33] and broken lines [34] of the hexagrams in the *Book of Changes*, the bones and flesh of the body, the rocks and water of the earth, just as they are male and female, day and night. The solid and broken lines compose a hexagram and give an explanation of a balancing of forces. Bones and flesh must be well proportioned in relation to one another. When all the elements are held in correct amounts, one obtains a rich structure from the combination. Any imbalances can be corrected by therapeutic intervention.

Chapter 6 of the *Lingshu* unites the qualities of vitality into four couples. If a life is to be lived to its end to accomplish the whole of its days, dictated by the endowments of its own nature and specific destiny, it

---

[31] The first Confucian virtue: authoritative personhood, humanness.

[32] Another great Confucian virtue: signification, a combination of righteousness and meaning.

[33] __ , hard.

[34] − − , soft.

depends upon the play of the soft *rou* 柔 and the hard *gang* 剛 , the weak *ruo* 弱 and the strong *qiang* 強 , the short *duan* 短 and the long *chang* 長 and finally, the *yin* 陰 and the *yang* 陽 .

For details we recommend that the reader undertake a deeper study of Chapter 6 of the *Lingshu*; here we simply state that the hard and the soft have a direct relationship to longevity and to premature death. The title given to Chapter 6 says it clearly: "The Hard and the Soft in Relation to Longevity or Premature Death" *shou yao gang rou* 壽夭剛柔 Chapter 6 of the *Lingshu* is concerned with showing the way life lasts by means of balanced and harmonious rapport at all levels: body and breath, skin and flesh, blood and breaths, and so on.

Lines 36 and 37 of our text (c. 187 · 226) show all the relationships between the breaths and between individuals (including sexual relationships), coming out of *yin/yang*. The hard/soft coupling stands for all the manifestations of *yin/yang*, whose good relationship prolongs life. "Corporeal" aspects are represented, but also strength and tenderness, the masculine and the feminine.

Jie 節 (to regulate) means to articulate the economy of life with correctness and firmness, and to maintain it within exact limits.

Tiao 調 (to balance) means to adjust and readjust in such a way that harmonious accord and true balance are obtained.

Acrobats and Tightrope-Walkers

This series of three injunctions in lines 32-37 of our text presents a significant sequence:

The first injunction (lines 32, 33) refers to a situation of celestial origin: the Four Seasons. Man has no choice but to conform to the natural and universal order they represent. The seasons are perceptible only through the variations of the breaths of Heaven recognized by man and by all beings. They show as cold and heat between Heaven and Earth. Our task is to adapt to cold and to heat climatically, and also to adapt within ourselves to cold and to heat.

The second injunction (lines 34, 35) refers to a situation of terrestrial origin. When the Great Clod of Earth, or each particular lump of clay that makes up the living, is moved by Heaven, internal stimulations are unleashed that let go and drop their breaths: it can be lively elation, or something that makes the breaths rise in a harsh counter current—

anger (cf *Suwen*, ch. 39, 62). It expresses itself in trees as the trembling caused by the spring breeze, or as the twisting of branches and leaves in a violent storm.

Only the human being can feel emotions, and only he can keep himself from reacting. He transforms the internal meteorological data into a harmonized breath, the absolute condition for his tranquillity. It is manifest when he is at rest, or standing, or sleeping, or seated, as well as when he is walking around or being active.

The third injunction (lines 36, 37) refers to a situation of life expressed by *yin/yang*. A particular human being is concerned with his own vitality or with that of a patient. He gauges the articulation and balance of the *yin* and the *yang*; he explores all the levels that his personal awareness and his diagnostic techniques can grasp. Then balance comes. It is obtained through meditation, through conduct of life (dietary, gymnastic, and other rules of living), and by acupuncture intervention that "re-balances." The patient is the product and the author of life's standards and of the conduct of the breaths and the meridians. The entire nomenclature of acupuncture and of the other techniques for life sweep through this gate.

Deflecting the Perverse Energies

The three examples of regulation presented to us are a triple development of knowing-how in action. If a being knows how to conduct his life as a function of the thirteen statements, he has an intimate grasp of his natural tendencies; he is acquainted with his nature, which is the outline of his organism and his psyche. He perceives the equilibrium and the movements of the forces around him and adapts spontaneously through his communion with Heaven, via the Spirits; he knows how to preserve and cultivate the subtle mechanism of life within himself. By following this path one already prevents and resolves the majority of illnesses.

Inadequacy vis-a-vis the external elements or, more seriously, between the elements that should constitute a being, unleashes discord and discomfort and lowers one's resistance to illness. To set each person back on his path is more valuable than prescribing a good remedy or piercing skin and flesh at proven points. Every needling, every therapy, must reorient the patient on this Way. That is the rooting of the Spirits: "In every needling, the method is above all to root oneself in the Spirits."

These three injunctions show us that the stability and the firmness of life's line, the permanent rooting in the Spirits, are nothing more than a perpetual changing, a permanent process of adaptation. It is a matter of adapting oneself to circumstances that are changeable because they are vital. And this applies not only to the conduct presented here, but beyond, to every therapeutic act. Every needling, every treatment, must also adapt to the situation presented by the patient. It is by looking at the Four Seasons or the explosions of joy and anger, that we can learn the tendencies of the person facing us. Then we can lead him into his own vital movement.

> In treating illness, *mai* 脉[35] and medicines have a primary importance that must not be neglected; but he who seeks to grasp the deep natural structure *li* 理 must, little by little, succeed in understanding the changes *yi* 易 ."
>
> *Zhang Jiebin*

In this way, having deflected the perverse energies, There will be long life and everlasting vision.
(lines 38, 39)

Those who have conducted themselves well will be led unerringly, if not without suffering, to the universalized term of their particular existence. The afterlife of each, beyond death, gives entrance into the "reunion of all beings." Each existence flows along to end at the "pond of tributaries," at the "Mysterious female from whose opening come Heaven and Earth." We must understand "knowing how to do" purely and simply as a "knowing how to be." From this solidity of the authentic within us flow out the extensions of our authenticity which are techniques, recipes, and arts. Right action is no more than a particular state of fullness of being of technicians, artisans, and artists of all kinds. Confucius knew the classics. He probably re-wrote them, more or less. A hundred thousand well-read scholars, of varying degree, followed him. One hundred thousand masters in all disciplines "divinely" practiced the liberal arts, and a hundred thousand more practiced professions that demanded equally authentic inspiration in detailing the one and only knowing-how. Bian the wheelwright hooped wheels perfectly without thinking about it;

---

[35] Network of animation, meridians, pulses.

another butchered beef without thinking about that either and without blunting his master-knife. Thus perfect bronzes have been cast since the Shang-yin dynasty (18th - 14th century B.C.). Also through intimate knowledge of knowing-how, in the kingdom of Chu they educated vain and arrogant princes, trained fighting cocks, tamed tigers without losing the tamer, raised greedy and disagreeable monkeys, and beat grasshoppers with sticks, without missing one.[36] From a unique and invisible source beginning simply in the moisture of earth and rocks are born the little rivulets that become, in every sense, the great rivers. There, in the minuscule, is the full power of "knowing how to be."

Long Life that procures everlasting vision may be assured only to the enlightened and courageous human who retains from all knowledge merely the knowing that equalizes doing and being. One could bow before such a pure representation of the outcome of all beings. Perhaps vision (where human activity is only a flashing glance) is the completion of a person's individual adventure. But many other lives will be lit from this flash for the same destiny: to see, to have vision.

---

[36] All of these anecdotes come from *Zhuangzi*.

Cascade II

General Organization of Chapter 8 of the Lingshu

This part of *Rooted in Spirit* is the completion of this study. The Great Acupuncturist is an artist and a wise person with a generous heart. The Tradition has initiated him into the mystery, and he stands before the door of all wonders. His hand is guided to the "places" of the body where the Spirits are rooted in the crossing of the breaths. This clever and helping hand is surrendered completely to the Spirits that dwell within the acupuncturist. His science is monumental, his dexterity supple, his touch like that of a blind musician, his heart makes magnanimous leaps. The movements of the needle receive their quality from all of this. The needle goes in to meet the breaths of a patient whose immediate condition and appearance have been recognized. To some degree this patient's essences have been deserted by the Spirits. The essences are affected by the imbalance of blood and breaths. The *yin/yang* rapport is disturbed. From external attacks that continue until they become internal attacks, or through an opening that awakens a rampant illness, breaths called excessive or deficient tend to establish themselves and create a pathological situation.

But all is not lost. The acupuncturist spoken of in the *Lingshu* will help you to disengage, by yourself, from your illness. He will assist you by "interrogating the nest, questioning the breath" (Victor Hugo, *Le Satyr*). He will reach the root of life where "newness and aliveness" arrive from moment to moment.

His hand sharpened and made precise by holding needles that he has chosen as a painter chooses his special brushes, the acupuncturist allows himself to be guided by his own Spirits. He calls Heaven and Earth to the points where their meeting gives birth to life. Thus the perverse breaths, whose sole purpose is to distort more and more, are driven away, and the regular, orthodox breaths can regather. The weakened essences that were ready to quit regain control of themselves. The Spirits that had left return, readjust the reins and do not spare the horses!

The patient forgets that he has been ill. He now basks in soft warmth and light. Liveliness bubbles up and pours forth. The person, healthy again, has a relaxed face, a restful manner, and a joyful expression. His step is alert, his gestures are quick but capable of restraint, his mind is lively but composed, his intent is sensible and open, and his will is ready for anything. The renewal of a living being is manifested by the radiance of his Spirits.

The complete teaching of this part of *Rooted in Spirit* can be presented thus:

> For every needling, the method above all is not to miss the rooting in the Spirits.[37]

---

[37] Lines 2, 3 (characters 1 · 83).

This being so, when there is apprehension and anxiety,
   worry and preoccupation attack the Spirits.   40
When the Spirits are attacked, under the effect of fear
   and fright,
There is a flowing out, there is a spilling over
   that cannot be stopped.

In a state of sadness and grief one is moved to the center.
There is a running dry and a stopping and life is lost.

Preyed upon by elation and joy, the Spirits are scared away
   and dispersed;   45
Hence there is no more thesaurization.

Preyed upon by oppression and sorrow, the breaths are
   closed and blocked;
Hence there is no more circulation.

Preyed upon by swelling anger, one is disturbed and led
   astray;
Hence everything is out of control.   50

Preyed upon by fear and fright, the Spirits are agitated
   and scared away;
Hence nothing can be contained any longer.

Characters 227 to 292

是 故 怵 惕 思 慮 者 傷 神
shi gu chu ti si lü zhe ze shang shen

神 傷 則 恐 懼 流 淫 而 不 止
shen shang ze kong ju liu yin er bu zhi

因 悲 哀 動 中 者 竭 絕 而 失 生
yin bei ai dong zhong zhe jie jue er shi sheng

喜 樂 者 神 憚 散 而 不 藏
xi le zhe shen dan san er bu cang

愁 憂 者 氣 閉 塞 而 不 行
chou you zhe qi bi sai er bu xing

盛 怒 者 迷 惑 而 不 治
sheng nu zhe mi huo er bu zhi

恐 懼 者 神 蕩 憚 而 不 收
kong ju zhe shen dang dan er bu shou

Structure of the Fragment (char. 227-292)

The parallelism in the construction delivers the meaning immediately. It is easy to isolate the pivotal points in the argument. Several clarifications are nonetheless useful:

a) To take charge of Beings is the function of the Heart, which fulfills this function with verve and joy. Things no longer work when apprehension turns into anxiety and worries become preoccupation. The normal movements of thought and reflection thus become a disturbance that deepens. This is the effect of the incessant stirring of a distressed heart. The Spirits are attacked by the disturbance. Protection of the heart — necessary to the acquisition of breaths for maintaining the essences — is no longer possible. Birds will not stay in a tree whose trunk and branches are being shaken.

b) Then essences and breaths start to "flow out and spill over" everywhere. One can retain nothing and one continues to be emptied indefinitely. "Fear" is a current of perverse breaths. It is like a mudslide that devastates one's vitality, and that nothing can stop.

c) Sadness and grief give repeated blows to the center of the being, in the place occupied by the heart. The vitality that resides there escapes, is depleted and runs dry, unable to again become a creative force and renewer of life.

d) Elation and joy are no less formidable. They have a disastrous effect on the Spirits, quick to be scared away and to flee. Their departure stops the vital process of thesaurization, and without thesaurization life is no longer possible.

e) Life can also be seen as a matter of the circulation of the breaths. All blockages of a certain length are dangerous and fatal. What is responsible for this? Melancholy and faintheartedness are responsible. They slow down, stop, and block the flow of breaths, causing the perversion of stagnation.

f) From another point of view life can be seen as the conducting of oneself with determination, suppleness and surety. This is governing oneself. One must see where one is going. Blind anger, rising powerfully, causes us to lose our way. We no longer govern anything, least of all ourselves.

g) Finally, to live means not being afraid to live. This nasty fear — whose hidden origin is apprehension turning to anxiety, and whose miry current drains and demolishes the deepest part of the being — is a direct threat to the Spirits. The Spirits in us are easily frightened; they have a great need for calm. If the Spirits could remain intimately permeated by the Essences, then merging with the most subtle of them, the Spirits would regather and would remain. But no, deathly fear strikes life in the heart, and the frightened Spirits abandon the shelter they had within us.

This being so, when there is apprehension and anxiety, worry and preoccupation attack the Spirits. (line 40)

"This being so" translates *shi gu* 是故 . *Shi* 是 is a demonstrative, used to recall what has just been said. *Gu* 故 names a circumstance. We translate: this being given, things being so, it follows that . . . .

A pathological situation that is going to be described flows out from the healthy situation that had been shown. Things now being thus (different and pathological), through the effect of anxious apprehension and worried preoccupation, the Spirits are attacked.

Apprehension and Anxiety

The intensity of the apprehension that turns into anxiety *chu ti* 怵惕 is variable and diversely manifested. This can simply be respectful, reverent fear, accompanied by a slight trembling movement of the body. Thus, in the *Book of History, Shujing,* we find apprehension and anxiety seizing a prince who has just been named king:

> Ah, I am incapable of the virtue I need, and now here I am
> heir to my predecessors, acceding to sovereign power! I
> tremble with terror in this extreme peril *chu ti.* I am awake
> at night, thinking of how I can avoid committing error.
> Couvreur, p. 372, revised translation

In the official Chinese history, princes show reverent fear. Does this fear go as far as trembling? The language is too conventional for us to be able to decide. So we must note that their anxiety robs them of sleep. It is better to admit that *chu ti* (apprehension and anxiety) expands to its strongest meaning, without necessarily having a pathological connotation.

In a famous text Mencius poses this principle: that seeing a child about to fall into a well, we are instinctively seized by apprehension and anxiety accompanied by an unavoidable shuddering. *Chu ti* is still the expression used. There is no pathology here either. Rather, we note the natural connection between the shuddering felt and the sight of imminent danger. The feeling is expressed normally by a change of attitude, an alteration of coloring (skin tone), of the voice, and of more internal sensations. Because of the unity of the vital movement, the organism reflects the distress signal produced originally in the heart.

Apprehension and anxiety *chu ti* may be passing states. In this case there is nothing seriously wrong within the person. But *chu ti* can move in and stay. Their negative effect is then propagated directly toward the Spirits through worry and preoccupation. The interior equilibrium is broken; a person no longer has peace; the luminous radiance of the Spirits dwindles imperceptibly until it is finally extinguished. The ground slips away from beneath a man who sees everything around him vacillating. The heart, life's operation center, no longer exercises its mastery. Apprehension and anxiety destabilize the individual, his thought, and his mind. The next stage of disintegration is panic, described by *Zhuangzi* in Chapter 21.

In this chapter two men challenge each other at archery. One of them, Baihun Wuren, is a Daoist adept; Yukou, the other, is a very proficient archer. The latter "stretched his bow with such a strong arm that he shot the arrow with a cup of water placed on his elbow, filled to the brim. As soon as an arrow was released the next was already in place. And during the entire time one would have thought him a statue." An artist! But Baihun Wuren leads him away from his usual shooting fields.

He takes him to the top of a mountain, to the edge of a dizzying peak. And Baihun Wuren places himself in shooting stance, his back to the abyss, his heels jutting out over the void. He invites his partner to come join him. And the latter, having lost all his means, is incapable of doing it. He dares not approach the edge of the precipice; he will never be able to shoot in this position, not even at the widest target. Then Baihun Wuren says to him:

> The supreme man *zhi ren* 至人 lifts his gaze toward azure Heaven, plunges it into the Yellow Springs, spreads it throughout to the Eight Poles *ba ji* 八極, and does so without alteration of his Spirits/breaths *shen qi* 神氣. But you tremble

with apprehension *chu* 怵 , and your eye cannot focus on anything. So it is with your innermost part *zhong* 中 ; it is in danger.

A man who is attacked by *chu ti* (apprehension and anxiety) when confronted by the unusual or by danger, is unable to hang on to the only reliable foundation: Azure Heaven, the Yellow Springs, the Eight Poles, that is to say, Heaven/Earth with its expanding median. He has not the strengh to entrust himself to his Heart and to the Spirits in his Heart. He undermines his own process of reaction that would have been able to get him out of this dangerous situation. He can only try to distance himself from the chasm. He does not succeed in taking charge of the beings, of ordering the events. How could his mind maintain itself correctly?

...worry and preoccupation attack the Spirits.
(line 40, continued)

The following couple, *si lü* 思慮 worry and preoccupation, manifests this internal degradation of the mind. *Si lü* is taken in a pejorative sense, inferred by the naming of the first couple, apprehension and anxiety *chu ti*.

With the couple *si lü* it is no longer a matter of thought that rings true, that spreads itself far and powerfully in an appropriate reflection, capable of organizing all the elements of a situation or a being, or of our own being. We have seen that apprehension and anxiety incapacitate once they are installed in the depths of the heart.

Thought *si* 思 and reflection *lü* 慮 are good, desirable, and useful when they are in the straight line of knowing-how *zhi* 智 ; then nothing escapes the greatness of the human spirit. This is affirmed by *Guanzi* (chapter *Xingshi*).

> When the thought and reflection *si lü* of a saint *sheng ren* (holy man) are in keeping with knowing-how *zhi*, there is nothing that is not within the range of his consciousness.

To have something in the heart—be it an idea, a thought, or a concern—is appropriate to man. But it is bad to transform thought into preoccupation and worry, or concern into obsession; it would be better to have an empty heart than a disturbed one. The Saint has neither preoccupation nor worry; he keeps himself in emptiness and pure serenity; he does not let ideas and reflections drone and proliferate.

Preoccupation and worry spoil the heart, just as colors spoil the eye and flavors spoil the mouth. We are the most profoundly perverted only by that with which we have a natural bond. Our heart, the location of thought, will be spoiled and disturbed by thoughts.

Chapter 8 of *Huainanzi* sets it out this way:

> When the luminous radiance of the Spirits *shen ming* is thesaurized [stored] within the Formless, and when the essences/spirits *jing shen* return to the Supreme Authenticity, then the eye is radiant and no longer oriented toward vision, the ear is fine and no longer just for hearing, the heart spreads out, is propagated far and wide, and is no longer for preoccupation and worry *si lü*.

The headache of worry and preoccupation *si lü* is an obstacle to the expansion of the heart, as vision limits the eyes and hearing the ears. Common use limits and de-natures their authentic use. For the eye is not simply made for seeing; it is made for radiating the light toward both the exterior and the interior. The ear is not simply made for hearing; it is also for receiving, taking, and understanding with finesse and discernment. The heart is not made simply to permit the germination of thoughts; it is there to dilate itself to the dimensions of Heaven/Earth. This is why no thought should occupy the heart, no worry should hold it back and shrink it.

In Chinese, to pay attention is to make one's heart very small *xiao xin* 小 心 . This is not diminishing it; it is making it subtle through sustained attention. Centering oneself and concentrating preserves the heart's nature, which is to be great and to be disposed to take charge of the totality of beings.

For thought and reflection to be free, balanced, and without preoccupation or worry, one's interior organization must function harmoniously. So states Chapter 1 of *Huainanzi*:

> Having established the free communication that permits the luminous radiance of the Spirits, one can come into possession of one's internal self. Thus, the exterior is mastered by the center, and the one hundred matters do not collapse. When the center has what it needs, then the

exterior is in a tempo of receiving/containing. When the center has what it needs, then the Five *Zang* are tranquil, and thought and reflection are well balanced.

But the five *zang* are not tranquil, the Spirits are not at peace, we do not have complete possession of ourself, of our actions and reactions; we are subject to apprehension and anxiety. In this state thought and reflection, which should show the way and lead to knowing-how, are out of balance, aggravating the situation. Led astray, the two-edged sword of thought and reflection turn against the one that shelters them, and they attack the Spirits in the heart. The individual is made ill by his own thoughts, by a caricature of his own reflection. His dispossession of himself increases through misuse.

It is not just a medical notion; a treatise as general as the *Lüshi Chunqiu* (Chapter 17) knows it:

> Through preoccupation and worry *si lü* one attacks oneself (through the heart). Knowing-how *zhi* goes off the track through excesses, and it is the loss of oneself.

The Spirits are attacked *shen shang* 神傷, the center of the personality is no longer under any control, and the personality itself no longer controls anything. Thoughts are like so many parasites on the sound waves, so many dissonances. We no longer hear the right note. Destabilized by apprehension and anxiety, we no longer know which Saint to devote ourselves to, which thought to entrust to ourselves again. If we could return to ourself, to the Spirits, to Heaven/Earth, we would escape degradation and would not lose ourself. But alas, it is impossible.

***When the Spirits are attacked, under the effect of
     fear and fright,
There is a flowing out, there is a spilling over
     that cannot be stopped*** *. (lines 41, 42)*

This way of being disoriented, shaken to one's foundation, unable to feel anything solid, resistant and sure — this is fear *kong* 恐 radiating into fright *ju* 懼.

Fear and fright are *kong ju* 恐懼.

Fear and fright are normal experiences. Wise dread and welcome prudence help one gauge the consequences of an action. The *Zhongyong* (*Unchangeable Milieu*, one of the Four Books of the Confucian school) says:

> For this reason the sage is watchful and pays attention, even when he sees nothing that calls for his vigilance; he is afraid and trembles (*kong ju*) even when he hears nothing that should frighten him. For him, the most important discovery is the secrets enfolded by his heart; and nothing but the tiniest signs will show. Thus he watches carefully over that which he alone knows (his thoughts and his most intimate feelings).
>
> Couvreur translation, p. 29

The timorous and fearful man of *Lingshu* Chapter 8 is not this sage. That man is incapable of penetrating himself; his interior is nothing more than the noise, the chaos that terrorizes him. His fear does not come to him so much from the exterior; it is an internal confusion, a disorganization of life, and an absence of the vital current, of joy and confidence in life.

The shaking that begins as just a quiver ends in near-total paralysis.

> Whereas small fears *xiao kong* 小恐 cause quivering, great fear *da kong* 大恐 paralyzes.
>
> *Zhuangzi*, Ch. 2, cf *Flutes et Champignons*

This is not the immobility wherein everything is contained; it is an absence of reaction and retention. One does not know where to turn; everything is collapsing and giving way; one knows neither where nor when to make the slightest stop; initiative has become impossible, and everything is slipping away; all seems irremediable and lost from the start.

Nothing is in its proper place; there is no cohesion or coherence of the *zang*, nor of the central *zang* which is the heart. The heart does not take its responsibility for being in charge; the Spirits can no longer shine and illuminate. Nothing reaches toward the heights, toward the light; all things come apart and leave. Everything flows out: tears and other bodily manifestations of those essences that are no longer retained.

In the beginning of *Cascade I*, (Heavenly) Virtue flowed out *de liu* to join with the (Earthly) breaths and give life, but here what is flowing out should be kept; this stream is perverse, hence the use of the character *yin* 淫 .[38]

Since the rooting in the Spirits is touched, the being no longer is rooted in the Spirits, no longer possesses himself, and it is impossible to stop *zhi* 止 the streaming-out that is the visible sensory mark of this perdition. Only recourse to the Spirits — the return of the Spirits — would arrest the flow and save the person. But that cannot be.

In Chinese the last words of line 42 ("cannot be stopped") can have a double meaning. "Without stopping" *bu zhi* 不止 could also mean that through the loss of essences, the Spirits are unable to stop, to establish themselves, or to remain in the individual.

In a state of sadness and grief one is moved to the center.
(line 43)

Sadness and grief are *bei ai* 悲哀

> At the death of his father, a son wept without interruption for three days; for three months he removed neither the arm band nor the hemp belt; for a year his thoughts were filled with profound feelings of sadness *bei ai* (he wept morning and night); his grief *you* 憂 lasted for three years.
> *Liji*, Couvreur II, p. 704, revised translation

Bei ai are thus the appropriate emotions felt by the "pious son" when encountering the death of a parent, especially of his father. This is public mourning, the emotion accompanying the definitive departure of the living being who gave you life.

The chapter "Questions on Mourning" (Chapter 32) of the *Liji* is full of considerations of sadness and grief *bei ai*; it describes the physical manifestations, the changes in external appearance, and the specific attitudes of a soul's mourning.

Examining the pairs of characters that express the feelings, one habitually brings up elation *xi* 喜 paired with anger *nu* 怒 , and similarly joy *le* 樂 paired sometimes with sadness *bei* 悲 , and sometimes with grief *ai* 哀 .

Sadness and grief *bei ai* are in opposition to the joy of life *le*, to the joy of Heaven, proper to all human life, that accepts itself and possesses itself. In a pathological sense, the movements and reactions implied by

---

[38] Something correct has been infiltrated, invested by perversion.

sadness and grief are in opposition to those implied by overflowing – even delirious – joy. The paragraphs commenting on lines 45 and 46 will elaborate upon the ravages of elation and joy when one "can no longer contain one's joy."

We have already noticed how sadness and grief strike repeated blows at the deep feeling of life, at the vivacity that is seeking to express itself and to rise and continuously free itself. Take mourning for a father: the text specifies one year's duration. To continue mourning, after the time is over, would be excessive. To wear mourning for oneself, to experience the feeling of loss of life when one is still alive, is a serious perversion. Life avenges itself and death is engendered by the mourning itself, for one has moved and shaken the internal; one has attacked the center of vitality.

This center *zhong* is, interchangeably, the five *zang* and their conjunctive action which thesaurizes the essences, frees the breaths, and lets itself be led by the Spirits. Similarly, the heart is the center: the center of the center, the dwelling place *par excellence* of the Spirits, the *shen*.

There is a running dry and a stopping, and life is lost. (line 44)

The freeing of the breaths stops, the essences are no longer thesaurized, and there is no renewal of vitality by the five *zang* or within them. There is no longer the least radiance. The luminous resonance of the shining world of the Spirits, which was reflected in and by each *zang*, no longer delights the being. All the warmth, the flame, all circulation and all peaceful lodging of this mysterious animating populace abandon each of these places (the *zang*) where life was joyously arrayed and fortified. The sober text does not forbid us to find how to re-make for ourselves both the enchanted feast of life that rises, and the poignant disenchantment of life that withdraws, runs dry, and finally stops.

The result of the sadness and grief is that life is lost *shi sheng* 失生 ; the *zang*, deprived of cohesion, no longer work symbiotically and synergistically; the heart is no longer sustained by the necessary heavenly joy; the taste for living is unraveled.

Let us return to this remarkable – but not ordinary –formula: life is lost *shi sheng*. What is lost is the capacity for what is in the dark to come into the light, for what is underground to come into the light of day. Bit by bit nothing sustains the vital spark any longer. There is no possibility of renewal.

Life denies the opposition of inside and outside, its only *raison d'être* being to live through all the smallest imaginable transformations until the death of sensory perception. We are not speaking of natural death when we evoke *shi sheng*, loss of life. We are speaking of the accepted, desired, sought-after wasting-away of a suicidal masochism.

To finish with this point, let us notice once more that neither here, nor in the parallel propositions that follow, do we say that the Spirits are attacked.

Preyed upon by elation and joy, the Spirits are
scared away and dispersed;
Hence there is no more thesaurization. *(lines 45, 46)*

Elation and joy are *xi le* 喜樂 .

In the normative sense of the expression, elation and joy *xi le* have already been studied (cf. *Secret Treatise of the Spiritual Orchid*[39]). Thus when *Shan zhong* 膻中 (the authority serving the heart, which stores, forms, and diffuses the breaths under the inspiration of the Spirits) accomplishes its charge fully, the result is elation and joy. Elation is vivaciousness and ease of circulation of breaths and blood; joy is the feeling of deep harmony that rules when the heart is healthy and well served, and when the Spirits open out at their leisure.

Normally, elation provokes expansion, movement toward the exterior, an externalization. With joy one leaps, thrills, and turns toward others even if they are strangers. Great joy can even stop the breath or make us roar. Do we not see it and hear it every day in the sports stadiums?

The *Treatise on Music (Yueji)*, found in the *Liji*, knows and analyzes these reactions:

> Music *yue* 樂 is composed of an ensemble of modulations *yin* 音 .[40] At its basis it has the feelings that are born in a man's heart under the influence of external objects.
>
> Thus when the heart is weighed down by grief *ai* 哀 (affliction), the sound is weak and soon ceases *sha* 殺 .
>
> When the heart is under the influence of happiness *le* (joy), the sound is full *dan* 嘽 and prolonged *huan* 緩 .

---

[39] Transcript of seminar by Claude Larre and Elisabeth Rochat de la Vallée, published by the British Register of Oriental Medicine, 1985.

[40] See the section entitled "When the Heart applies itself, we speak of Intent" (line 26) for the analog between modulation *yin* 淫 , and intent *yi* 意 .

> When the heart experiences a sudden and passing joy *xi*
> (elation), the sound suddenly takes off, *fa* 發, and is scattered
> far and wide *san* 散 .
> When the heart is moved by anger *nu* 怒, the voice be-
> comes turgid and the tone is caustic . . .
>
> Couvreur translation, Liji, II, p. 46

As we have seen, grief comes close to putting someone to death *sha*; its movement is contrary to the leaping forth of life seen in the springtime.

There are strong analogies between this passage of *Liji* and our text of *Lingshu* Chapter 8 concerning elation and joy. The character *dan* 嘽, meaning fullness of sound, is similar to the one used in *Lingshu* 8 for "scaring away" *dan* 憚, with only a change of the radical. That of the heart 心 is more appropriate in the context of emotions, but it looks quite similar to the other.

According to Wieger (Etymological Lesson 72E), the etymology of *dan* 單 is "to attack someone with cries 叫 and a pitchfork 草 ." It is a matter of excitation, of an attack that is certainly going to cause someone or something to flee.

By varying the radicals and conserving the same graphic phonetic group 單, ideograms are obtained with the following meanings: to dust, to chase dust with an instrument 撣 ; to fear, to recoil before 憚 ; to strike with small repeated blows 彈 ; to stir up the fire 燀 ; to spread out and develop 闡 ; to combat, to fight 戰 ; and with the radical for spirits 示 , the double meaning of the ideogram *shan* 禪 meaning to abdicate or to contemplate.

With the mouth 口 in the case of music, or with the heart 心 in the case of feelings, *dan* 單 is an aggressive stimulation that pushes to the outside.

For diffusion (to spread oneself far and wide) or for dispersion (head-long flight), the ideogram is the same in both *Lingshu* Chapter 8 and in the *Liji*: *san* 散 . Diffusion is healthy; dispersion is pathological. In the latter case, the inside empties itself, there is dilapidation toward the exterior. The ongoing recklessness of joy causes a person to lose all notion of danger or of simple restraint. Nothing is kept or saved. But far from being real generosity, this is only useless waste; the forces of life – essences and breaths – are driven outside the body by this tendency toward exteriorization (to go toward the exterior, the appropriate movement of summer) (cf. *The Way of Heaven*). But following behind

the essences and breaths are the Spirits themselves, left without support or echo, flurrying about like scared sparrows.

In the ancient world the Spirits are birds (cf *Bannière Funéraire de
Mawangdui*). The Spirits have the freedom of flight. They are also
fragile birds, easily startled or frightened. A lively stimulation *xi* or a
boundless expansion *le* is like a mad dog terrifying the barnyard or the
child or the bird; stirred up among themselves, they scatter.

If everything is pushed outside, how can the essences continue to
be thesaurized in the interior? If, scared away, the Spirits are dispersed, how can the *zang* still thesaurize?

Perverse situations reinforce their harmful effects; thesaurization
becomes impossible. There is loss of life, not because the taste or the
feeling for living has disappeared, but simply because there is no more
thesaurization.

Finally let us notice that it is the feelings most specifically attached
to the heart — elation and joy — that cause the *zang* 臟 to lose their
natural property of thesaurization *cang* 藏 .

Preyed upon by oppression and sorrow, the breaths are closed and blocked; Hence there is no more circulation. *(Lines 47, 48)*

Oppression and sorrow are *chou you* 愁憂

You 憂 is grief that overwhelms, a fright that is a suffering, and
an oppression that causes discomfort and embarrassment. All of this
fatigues and slows things down, causing blockages and difficulties
with circulation, a sinking, a melancholy immobility.

Chou 愁 is a distressing contraction; the heart tightens and becomes rigid.
All that is gathered in the heart moves no more; sadness imprints everything.

Notions of hindrance and discomfort predominate. Whatever other
feelings one experiences (and there are many coupled with *you*), the
oppression cannot leave. An extenuating despondency makes the feet
drag and all circulation stop dead. Everything responsible for the
circulation is touched by a profound melancholy, by this vital obstacle.

The center and the roundhouse of communications is always the
heart. It is not content to merely circulate the blood and send the
breaths as messengers; it sends the Spirits. Its emptiness permits the
free play of emotions, the transformations permitting the balancing of
the passions. The heart may also be attacked by oppression and sorrow
chou you. The expression *you xin* 憂心, a heart overwhelmed with

sorrow, is common in the *Book of Odes (Shijing)*. The *Neijing* indicates this coming together several times:

> Under the blow of oppression and sorrow *chou you*, of preoccupations and worry *si lü*, the heart is attacked. . . .
>
> *Suwen*, Chapter 73

> Oppression and sorrow *chou you*, fear and fright *kong ju*, take the attack to the heart.
>
> *Lingshu*, Chapter 4

> In the case of preoccupation and oppression *si you*, all of the heart's connections *xin xi* 心繫 tighten *ji* 急.; the heart's system *xin xi* being tight, the "ways" of the breaths *qi dao* are closed off *yue* 約 ; and being closed off, there is no more ease *bu li* 不利 ."
>
> *Lingshu*, Chapter 28

> Obstruction and blockage *ge sai* 隔塞, closure and interruption *bi jue* 閉絕, high and low are no longer in free communication *tong* 通 , and thus there is the illness called "violent oppression" *bao you* 暴憂.
>
> *Suwen*, Chapter 28

And finally, in Chapter 48 of *Lingshu*:

> When the heart is small, it is easily attacked by oppression *you* 憂.

How can the heart expand and be large under the constraint of oppression? Inversely, a heart that is small by nature has a predisposition to feel small, tight, uncomfortable: in short, to be in a state of oppression. The entire psyche of the individual will be marked by it throughout his life.

One might believe that such prostration and oppression are accompanied only by sadness and grief. This is not so; they can be coupled with something that seems antithetical — anger. Thus, in *Lingshu*, Chapter 66:

> One is brutally attacked by external cold, and if one is attacked internally by oppression and anger *you nu* (anger full of oppression, that suffocates), then the breaths rise in a counter-current. When the breaths rise in a counter-current,

then the six *shu* 輸 [41] are no longer in free communication, and the warming breaths no longer circulate. . . .

This makes us think of a kind of anger turned inward, one that does not explode but blocks all circulation, including respiration.

Here, in the expression *chou you* 愁憂 , what reinforces this distressing oppression is the gathering, contracting, and drawing in of autumn. No more unfurling. Nothing is more contrary to the heart and to its free Spirits. No more circulation. And this means circulation of blood, breath, and also Spirits.

Preyed upon by swelling anger, one is troubled and led astray;
Hence everything is out of control. *(lines 49, 50)*

Anger that becomes inflated is *sheng nu* 盛怒 .

Worse than a great anger *da nu* 大怒 [42] is anger that does not stop rising. Again one abandons oneself and empties one's life out. But this time it is not through powerless leakages, or by a drying up of the source of life, or even by blockages, but by a violent and continual propulsion that amplifies itself, that hurls and projects the *yin* toward the *yang*, thrusts everything upward and outward, and transports everything into an exaggeration of the vital momentum and of the *yang* movement in an excited fit of anger that feeds on itself.

The *yin* leaves via the *yang*: *yin chu zhi yang* 陰出之陽; in this malady one is easily angered and is not cured *bu zhi* 不治 .[43]

Suwen, Chapter 23

Letting everything be transported by an unbridled *yang*, we allow ourselves to be carried away and allow our interior – the intimate vitality, the individual – to be carried away. We are led astray; nothing is structured, rooted, or correctly oriented any longer within the mind, the

---

[41] The different points that act specifically at a distance, from the meridian to the interior organ; for example, the points we call the five elemental points.
[42] cf *Suwen*, Chapter 3.
[43] One does not control oneself.

thoughts, or the emotions. It is a complete rout. We are no longer in control *bu zhi*, whether speaking of the therapist's control in trying to heal her patient, or of the control each person must exercise over himself.

> The year of great overtaking by Wood: when it is intense, one has no discernment and becomes angered easily *hu hu shan nu* 忽.忽.善怒
>
> Suwen, Chapter 69

As with elation and joy, all that should remain in place to be thesaurized by the *zang* is uprooted from the internal zones.

With anger that swells, we emphasize the violence of the process and the rising of the phenomenon. Elation (lively joy) becomes less intense as it moves away from its beginning. But anger feeds on itself if not regulated or tempered, or if blindness or the lack of discernment prevents reason. Elation and joy attack the Spirits directly, disturbing them and causing them to flee. Anger empties the *yin* (cf *Suwen*, Chapter 5) and inflames itself, becoming very *yang*. One can no longer be anchored in profound reality; judgment no longer exists, but there is insane conduct, the loss of one's way and loss of control. It is the opposite of the function of the Liver as defined in *Suwen*, Chapter 8 (cf *Secret Treatise of the Spiritual Orchid*): to be the general of the armies who gives forth an exact analysis and sensible reflection.

Military treatises, such as the *Sunzi bingfa* (*The Art of War*, by Sunzi), offer good examples of one's being led astray, which can strike either the general in charge or the superior officers. Thus a general who becomes angry will no longer follow the plans and projects that he had established after a detailed analysis of the circumstances. He will march on the enemy without taking his plans into account, manifesting in his orders and positions the disorder that rules him internally. Similarly, superior officers who are full of wrath and blinded by fury, no longer even listen to their orders, but throw themselves into combat without taking into account what is possible and what is not, or what will be the probable outcome of the battle. All that counts for them is blow for blow, the disorderly and useless strike that leaves them exhausted and distraught.

Thus Huainanzi can write:

> Violence *nu* (anger) is to go in a counter-current against virtue *de*.

All kinds of conduct that it serves us to adopt are presented in *The Book of the Way and the Virtue (Daodejing)*, from which Huainanzi never deviates. The teaching of Chapter 68 can be recalled usefully here, taking care not to limit to military art alone a general directive of reserve, prudence, avoidance, and awareness of the "low" side that accompanies the manifestation of Virtue:

> Who knows how to be a war chief is not bellicose,
> Who knows how to lead combat does not give in to anger,
> Who knows how to triumph does not confront his adversary,
> Who knows how to handle men humbles himself before them.

Preyed upon by fear and fright, the Spirits are agitated and scared away; Hence nothing can be contained any longer. *(lines 51, 52)*

Fear and fright *kong ju* 恐懼 have already appeared in lines 41, 42: " . . . under the effect of fear and fright/There is a flowing out. . . ."

In their first appearance, fear and fright were mentioned after the attack aimed at the Spirits by apprehension and anxiety, by worry and preoccupation *chu ti si lü* 怵惕思慮. In this second occurrence, fear and fright will cause the agitation that scares away the Spirits.

The scaring away of the Spirits *dan* 憚 is also another refrain; we have already seen it as the expression of the harmful effect of elation and joy.

These refrains point out that this last proposition, while having its own value, also serves as conclusion for the ensemble of characters 227-292.

It specifies that the blow to the Spirits has repercussions upon the essences: the Spirits are scared away and full of agitation; it is the opposite of the peace they should enjoy without ceasing. Being thus agitated and frightened, the Spirits are no longer watched over and, in turn, can no longer keep guard. Nothing is held onto, and the essences themselves, unable to take advantage of any retention, are incapable of being seized, gathered, welcomed, or renewed. What is challenged here is fidelity to oneself via the renewal of the essences (according to their model), and the guarding of the Spirits. Not only are the Spirits frightened, but the pure essences which could hook them, retain and calm them, are at the point where they can no longer be received, assimilated, or guarded by the being.

It is a question of the development of the first proposition. Fear and fright, already resulting in a blow to the Spirits, only aggravate the situation, marked already by the frightening away of the Spirits and the loss of internal thesaurization.

What is the difference between the stoppage of thesaurization *bu cang* 不藏 of the essences, which occurs when elation and joy distract us from this fundamental life-maintenance process, and the above-mentioned loss of ability to contain *bu shou* 不收 the essences?

Thesaurization is the active guarding of the refined essences of the organism for the releasing of the correct and authentic breaths. To contain is to retain at all levels of the organism; to be able both to introduce and to assimilate, as in alimentation, and also to retain all aspects of vitality that take form within a being. The essences referred to are the models for renewal and the very materials of this renewal.

Three Readings

The simplicity and clarity of a classical text are such obvious qualities that sufficient attention is not always brought to the fact that the texts lend themselves to slightly differing readings, according to the way one interprets them and determines their organizational structures. It is not enough to point out a large number of verbal symmetries with the regular returning of syntactic points of articulation from which every-thing arranges itself neatly and harmoniously. We must still consider that several structures can be proposed, without any one imposing itself absolutely, or without any one being too improbable. For this fragment (c. 227-292) we will take three layouts that have the merit of being compatible, and each of which can legitimately enrich our perception of the profundity of the text's vital inspiration.

First Reading: Six Statements

This breakdown seems the most obvious. It is the one we have adopted for the presentation of the preceding commentaries. In addi-tion, the end of Chapter 8 of *Lingshu* repeats the totality in six

---

[44] A seventh-century compilation by Yan Shangshan, presenting and commenting upon texts, of which the majority belong to the *Neijing*.

[45] A fragment of line 41 ("attack the Spirits") and all of line 42.

explanatory paragraphs (c. 528 - 644, lines 100-120). The *Taisu* version,[44] suppressing in particular characters 234 -241,[45] presents six strictly paralleled statements.

Whether the ideogram for the Spirits *shen* 神 is repeated or not, the trouble is indisputably a question of a disturbance that touches the Spirits, because the disturbance has its origin in the heart of the individual, in the center of his or her life.

The center of life is the heart that takes on the burden of all beings. The heart can also be considered as the unity of the Five *Zang*. The five *zang* are the receptacles of the Spirits under different modalities, all capable of being mixed with the heavenly Spirits, which dwell most appropriately in the heart, the sovereign of the person and that which constitutes the sovereign person. The mystery of the knot of life is established in a relationship "by Five" (multiplied by five), whose effects are manifested according to the relationship "by Six." That which works "by Five" produces the Breaths (cf. *Suwen*, Chapter 5). The effects produced, and their system, are led by Six. Thus we say that Heaven has Six Breaths and man has Six Qualities of Breaths (cf. *Suwen*, Chapter 6). The Five is revealed in the Six.[46]

"Five" represents the constition of a center, where the Breaths of different qualities (this differentiation symbolized by "Four," the Four Seasons) are joined together in an association that is powerful and forever changing. This center permits the vital thrust and, above all, the organization of the vital thrust. "Six" represents the result of this internal organization in a network of relationship and circulation. The different qualities of Breaths that constitute a Being and a life are regularly distributed for nourishing, maintaining, defending, and rebuilding the entire space in which life unfolds. For a human, that space is the body; for the cosmos, it is the Universe inside the "Six Junctions" (the four directions in space, plus the zenith and the nadir). Thus man has Five *Zang* and Six Qualities of Breaths expressed by the Six Great Meridians, just as in the Universe life is produced by the Five Elements

---

[46] In Chinese numerology, Dao, or Heaven (i.e. the Unique power sustaining all of life), is One. So that things do not remain as they are, in a static state, another number is introduced: One becomes Two (*yin/yang* or Heaven/Earth). In comes Man to create dynamic movement between Heaven and Earth (Three: Heaven/Earth/Man). Next, Four Seasons develop, expanding into seasons in Heaven and climates or directions on Earth. To move Four from a fixed position, Five appears as a center around which Four can begin to rotate. The process continues, with something new being revealed by each succeeding Number. Every Number or condition requires the next one in order for the life of the Universe to continue in movement on all of its levels.

and maintained by the Six Breaths. It is this fundamental organization of a network of distribution depending upon a balanced and tranquil Center that is disburbed when emotions and passions break the serenity and equilibrium.

In characters 227 · 292 (lines 40-52) six statements reveal the disturbance of the Spirits resulting from one's being a victim of the preoccupation and worry that are born in a heart gnawed at by apprehension and anxiety, or being prey to the sadness and grief that undermines the foundation of the vital thrust, or being victimized by delirious excitement, or by deep melancholy, or by growing irritability, or finally, if all the foundations of the being are wavering, by fear and fright.

There is another symmetry of six here. Each of the six statements naming the disturbance by a powerful emotion is followed by a statement naming the negative result, making a matching total of six negative consequences: no more stopping *bu zhi* 不止 ; loss of life *shi sheng* 失生 ; no more thesaurization *bu cang* 不藏 ; no more circulation *bu xing* 不行 ; no more control *bu zhi* 不治 ; no more containment *bu shou* 不收.

The *Taisu* does not say: "no more stopping" *bu zhi*, but "no more solidity" *bu gu* 不固 . With everything escaping and overflowing, there is no longer that solid holding of life that must be guaranteed for the (safety of the) interior (cf *Suwen*, Ch. 3).

The only apparent flaw of symmetry would be "loss" of life *shi sheng* 失生 , all the other results being introduced by the negative *bu* 不 . This causes no problem in the style of classical Chinese, however.

Second Reading: Seven Statements

The division of the text into seven statements does not require the suppression of characters 234 · 241. (see footnote 45)

1) This being so, when there is apprehension and anxiety, worry and preoccupation attack the Spirits. *(line 40)*

2) When the Spirits are attacked, under the effect of fear and fright, There is a flowing out, there is a spilling over that cannot be stopped. *(lines 41, 42)*

3) In a state of sadness and grief one is moved to the center. There is a running dry and a stopping and life is lost. *(lines 43, 44)*

4) Preyed upon by elation and joy, the Spirits are scared away and dispersed;
Hence there is no more thesaurization. *(lines 45, 46)*

5) Preyed upon by oppression and sorrow, the breaths are closed and blocked:
Hence there is no more circulation. *(lines 47, 48)*

6) Preyed upon by swelling anger, one is disturbed and led astray;
Hence everything is out of control. *(lines 49, 50)*

7) Preyed upon by fear and fright, the Spirits are agitated and scared away;
Hence nothing can be contained any longer. *(lines 51, 52)*

The first three propositions are of about equal length (10, 10, and 11 characters); the following four are a bit shorter (9, 9, 8, and 9 characters).

The first proposition contrasts with the context immediately preceding, at the end of Cascade I:

> Thus knowing-how is the maintenance of life. . . . "In this way, having deflected the perverse energies/There will be long life and everlasting vision." (characters 187 - 226, lines 31-39)

But too often this is what happens:

1) One has not been able to maintain his life; he has not fulfilled his responsibilities; he has allowed himself to form tendencies (tendencies which in this case could be *zhi* 志, will) contrary to the development and the flowering of human nature within him. He has forgotten the dignity, the grandeur, and the celestial quality of the Spirits, which are the heavenly mandate. All those who go against nature, against the plan of harmonious development, strike blows against that part of themselves that is the guarantor and guide of the heavenly outcome – the Spirits.

By a fearful letting-go, by an undoing of the normal internal tension, by a lack of courage to face both oneself and situations or beings, by having allowed preoccupations and invasive worries to seep into the self, the individual has caused the Spirits to be attacked. They no longer radiate outward; no longer do they reach far. The Heaven within is renounced by conduct that offends its majesty.

2) When the vital tension is slackened, and once the solidity of a life well-anchored in the Spirits is weakened, there is a total sinking, a

general relinquishing that manifests in the form of lost liquids and drained essences. That which forms us is allowed to be lost.

3) Sadness and grief double the blows against the internal, intimate center. If this center is rendered incapable of fulfilling its task of vital maintenance which is divided between the five *zang*, there is drying up, cessation, and then loss of the vital surge. Life dries up at its source, in the *zang*, the vital center of man.

4) Ravaged by externals, due to too much elation and joy, the Spirits are scared away and neither guarded nor thesaurized. The physical impression is one of "spiritual malaise." The individual loves excitement, but the Spirits do not find their happiness there.

5) Blockage, on the inside as well as the outside, causes an interruption of the circulation of the breaths as a result of oppression or of prostration that compresses all expansion and expression of vitality and vivacity.

6) The rise in power of "anger" provokes the breaths to be led astray. Anger blinds; useful conduct of life is no longer possible.

7) Fear and dread cause the Spirits to be agitated and scared away; one can no longer gather them in, and one no longer has anything to gather in. This last proposition is the end of a process; it serves as the conclusion while recalling the first proposition.

This organization by seven conforms to the numerological value of the emotions (there are seven emotions). The relationship of the Spirits to the essences is expressed by the number Seven (cf. especially Chapter 7 of *Huainanzi*, called *jing shen* 精神, essences/Spirits: the subtle and light spirits that are produced by the essences, and which preserve their quality).

The first statement in line 40 ("when there is apprehension and anxiety, worry and preoccupation attack the Spirits") puts the disturbance at the highest level of spiritual life. From our interior world we slide towards the second proposition, presenting evidence of the transformation of anxious apprehension into fear and fright, commotions that are already farther inside the organism.

The final proposition (number 7) sketches an inverse stylistic movement: we see how fear and fright act upon the Spirits which become agitated and alarmed. It is a precise description of the situation of the Spirits in their terrain (a living being's heart). Here *shang* (to attack) and *dang* (agitated) come together: the first proposition expresses an attack on the Spirits; the last shows this attack as agitation.

Shang 傷 , to attack. This can be at the heavenly level, which we may confuse (wrongly) with the abstract plane, whereas it is the power of life, absolutely real and concrete (but imperceptible to the senses), that can be reached only by the Art of the Heart, by sacrifice, by prayer, by worship of the ancestors, and by remembering one's own heavenly origin.

Dang 蕩 , to be stirred up or agitated, is located at the bodily level, fully exercised in the concrete existence we experience every day.

Dan 憚 , scared away, alarmed, fearful. The reader can hesitate between two aspects of the meaning of this — one turned toward fear, the other toward suffering. It is better to join the two aspects, presenting an upset of the heart that paralyzes all activity. Certainly that is the meaning. One can no longer draw out that which is necessary for life. One can no longer seek support for a "dying life." The whole context leans toward this interpretation. The breaths that, through the essences, normally live under the inspiration of the Spirits, trickle out in futile and pernicious agitation. Vitality becomes scarce; no longer concentrated, it is dissipated and dispersed. One can no longer retain either the breaths or the Spirits, because there are no longer essences for maintaining life.

Third Reading: Two Groups

This is a refinement of the preceding grouping. We can discern two groups within the seven propositions: the first three propositions (Group A); and the last four propositions (Group B).

Group A) The first three propositions represent attacks on the Spirits which are troubled, weakened, and tormented. They no longer hold themselves together, nor can they seem to hold on to life; everything is adrift in the current, and nothing can stop the process. One loses one's joy in living, the taste for life, the pleasure of existing. There is a sickening (*taedium vitae*), a taste for death. The ritual sentiment of mourning inhabits the heart and clothes the Spirits. The harmonics that compose life are dissolved: life is lost; the water in the vase leaks out drop by drop; one's being is broken.

This is the ineluctable process whereby the tone of the Spirits and the tone they give to the being color and darken life until its fatal end. One empties oneself without desiring to retain anything, without stopping oneself. One lets everything go, losing one's vitality, until life is lost.

We can distinguish three stages corresponding to the three statements.

First, there is the heavenly aspect of the attack on the Spirits. Are the Spirits not Heaven tucked away inside us?

Second, there is the earthly aspect of spilling and flowing out. The metaphor of liquid, of essences that flow out, bring to our minds the Earth, clay, and all that gives form.

Third, there is the median aspect *zhong* 中 . This median, emerging in man, is moved, stirred up, and turned upside down. This median *zhong* is man, the interior of man who forms his existence through the *zang*. *Zhong* can be man living between Heaven and Earth, seen as that which produces life in its deepest aspect. A median always shelters another more intimate median, and on and on indefinitely. In the case of serious disturbance, the heart of the median — there where the formed being shows on the surface — is attacked. "There is weeping without reason in this disheartened heart" (Paul Verlaine, *Romance Sans Paroles*).

Group B) The second group, consisting of the last four propositions, is the more descriptive part. It divides into Four Poles the effects of the loss of the center presented in Group A. This is not the place to suggest an assimilation of the four aspects (these four breaches of the actions that protect life), with the Four Seasons and the Four Orientations. However, we can believe that in the era that these texts were written, it was normal to explain and expand "by four" a situation that was already expressed on three levels and centered around an axis.

(1) Nothing is actively retained inside any longer;

(2) Nothing circulates correctly any longer;

(3) Nothing is rhythmic or controlled any longer;

(4) Nothing, in short, is held, contained, or retained.

The next portion (characters 293-463) of *Lingshu* Chapter 8, which takes up lines 40-52 and explains them, links the two erring ways of Group A (no more stopping, and loss of life) to the heart and liver, whereas the four dysfunctions of Group B are linked to the lung, spleen, and kidneys (and essences). Thus in Group A the deviation of the two masculine *zang* is exposed, corresponding to the *yang* seasons and to the rising of life; in Group B the deviation of the *yin* feminine *zang* is exposed.

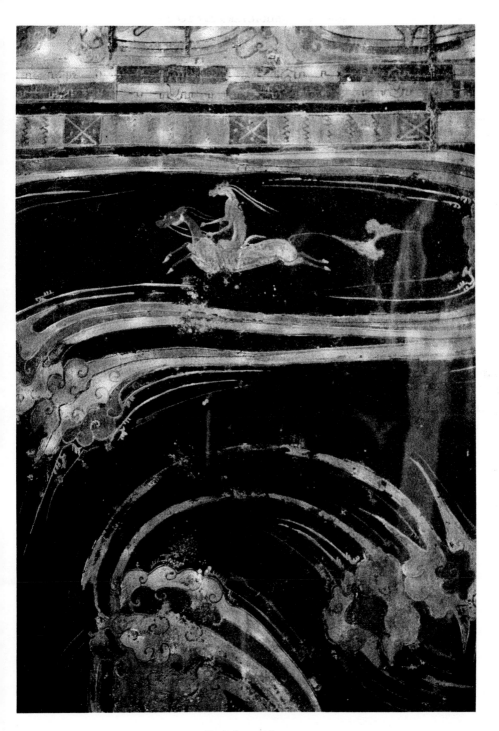

Spirits (Shen)

When the Heart falls prey to apprehension and anxiety, to
worry and preoccupation,
The Spirits are attacked.
When the Spirits are attacked, under the effect of fear and
fright, one loses possession of oneself,   55
The well-developed forms become emaciated, and the mass
of flesh is ravaged.
The body hair becomes brittle and one has all the signs of
premature death.
One dies in winter.

When the Spleen falls prey to oppression and sorrow and
cannot free itself,
The Intent is attacked.   60
When the Intent is attacked, one is disturbed until the
disorder is total,
The four limbs can no longer rise.
The body hair becomes brittle and one has all the signs of
premature death.
One dies in spring.

When the Liver falls prey to sadness and grief, one is
moved in one's center,   65
The *Hun* are attacked.
When the *Hun* are attacked, one loses reason and becomes
forgetful; there is no vitality.
Without vitality one cannot guarantee the norm.
In this situation where the *yin* apparatus contracts, where
the musculature cramps,
The flanks on both sides can no longer rise.   70
The body hair becomes brittle and one has all the signs of
premature death.
One dies in autumn.

Characters 293 to 463

心 怵 惕 思 慮 則 傷 神
Xin chu ti si lü ze shang shen

神 傷 則 恐 懼 自 失
shen shang ze kong ju zi shi

破 胭 脫 肉
po jun tuo rou

毛 悴 色 夭 死 於 冬
mao cui se yao si yu dong

脾 愁 憂 而 不 解 則 傷 意
Pi chou you er bu jie ze shang yi

意 傷 則 悗 亂 四 肢 不 舉
yi shang ze men luan si zhi bu ju

毛 悴 色 夭 死 於 春
mao cui se yao si yu chun

肝 悲 哀 動 中 則 傷 魂
Gan bei ai dong zhong ze shang hun

魂 傷 則 狂 忘 不 精
hun shang ze kuang wang bu jing

不 精 則 不 正 當 人
bu jing ze bu zheng dang ren

陰 縮 而 攣 筋 兩 脅 骨 不 舉
yin suo er luan jin liang xie gu bu ju

毛 悴 色 夭 死 於 秋
mao cui se yao si yu qiu

When the Lung falls prey to boundless elation and joy,
The *Po* are attacked.
When the *Po* are attacked, one loses reason.   75
With this loss of reason, the Intent knows no one,
The skin shrivels and wrinkles.
The body hair becomes brittle and one has all the signs of
    premature death.
One dies in summer.

When the Kidneys fall prey to anger that swells without
    stopping,   80
The Will is attacked, one can no longer even remember
    what one has just said,
The loins and dorsal spine can neither lean forward nor
    lean backward,
Neither bend, nor straighten.
The body hair becomes brittle and one has all the signs of
    premature death.
One dies in the last stage of summer.   85

Under the effect of fear and fright from which one cannot
    free oneself,
The Essences are attacked, the bones grow stiff, impotence
    leads to withdrawal.
At times the Essences descend by themselves.

Characters 293 to 463 (cont.)

肺喜樂無極則傷魄
Fei xi le wu ji ze shang po

魄傷則狂
po shang ze kuang

狂者意不存人皮革焦
kuang zhe yi bu cun ren pi ge jiao

毛悴色夭死於夏
mao cui se yao si yu xia

腎盛怒而不止則傷志
Shen sheng nu er bu zhi ze shang zhi

志傷則喜忘其前言
zhi shang ze xi wang qi qian yan

腰脊不可以俯仰屈伸
yao ji bu ke yi fu yang qu shen

毛悴色夭死於季夏
mao cui se yao si yu ji xia

恐懼而不解則傷精
Kong ju er bu jie ze shang jing

精傷則
jing shang ze

骨酸痿厥
gu suan wei jue

精時自下
jing shi zi xia

When the Heart falls prey to apprehension and
   anxiety, to worry and preoccupation,
The Spirits are attacked.
When the Spirits are attacked, under the effect of
   fear and fright, one loses possession of oneself,
The well-developed forms become emaciated, and the
   mass of flesh is ravaged.
The body hair becomes brittle and one has all the
   signs of premature death.
One dies in winter. (lines 53-58)

Lingshu Chapter 8 continues by looking at each of "six situations." In each (except in the last case), a *zang* is indicated as being specifically attacked. This done, there is a brief mention of the physical symptoms which announce, by their presence, the specific disturbance that has occurred in the invisibility within the subject. There is always the belief that nothing happens internally that does not ultimately appear at the perceptible and palpable level.

Up until now, in the first thirteen lines of the second part of *Lingshu* Chapter 8 (lines 40-52), we have discovered the attacks upon and the emotional tendencies within the Center, that is, within the heart and within the Spirits of the heart. We know the reason: the heart takes responsibility for, takes on and masters all the feelings; the Spirits inspire them (the feelings); their peaceful equilibrium is necessary for life to be powerful throughout and constantly regenerated.

In the "reprise" that constitutes the next thirty-six lines, and which we are now examining, things are seen more closely. The Center is split along Five axes, and then there is a sixth situation. The Center is broken open to permit the therapist an approach specific to each of its constituents, and to allow the specific treatment that will be effective. This does not exclude the possibility that health may be restored simply by the powerful irradiating presence of a great master, without needing a specific diagnosis or treatment; but masters like this are not found on every street corner.

More commonly, the therapist, after having seen which aspect of the vital movement is attacked, re-balances the whole by treating the specific breakdown that he knows with certainty because of the character-istic symptoms present in the patient.

The treatment is not narrowly or reductively "symptomatic," how-ever. Nor should we say, for example, in the name of who-knows-what vague psychosomatism, that anxiety and worries cause weight loss. This is not necessarily false, but neither is it absolutely true. The reasoning is, rather, that the patient is disturbed in one of the sectors of his or her activity, because one of the five important emotional aspects corresponding to a *zang* (each of which, in turn, represents one of the Five Elements) is out of order. The practitioner discerns the origin of the problem and is concerned about its spreading from that starting point. When a movement is disturbed at its source, that is, in its deepest tendencies (in the special acts of the will-to-live, and in the Spirits that animate and permanently create each *zang*), bit by bit the axis of life is subjected to a disturbance whose visible signs can be tracked, and from which the most deeply hidden irregularities can be inferred. Around the axis of the disease or the illness, the interference of all the axes develop perverse effects. This is expressed by the "control cycle" *(ke)*,[47] when the control becomes pathological.

When one falls prey to apprehension and anxiety, doubled by worry and preoccupations, the central vital movement—that which is summed up, centered, and deployed in and by the heart—is involved. How, in this state, can a lively circulation or a healthy flourishing be furthered? The attack is upon the deepest treasure of the heart, upon its Spirits, which allow the heart to be master of circulation and of the flourishing of the Being.

In this case, the fire shining in the heart is now only a weak ember, incapable of really animating anything. Animation (for example, through the networks of animation: the *mai* or the blood) goes slack. The movement of the heart, of the fire that draws upward, is weakened; the power of life flags; and the essences are no longer correctly and firmly held. Everything runs out, as in spermatorrhea.

---

[47] The control *(ke)* cycle is a balancing cycle within the Five Elements wherein, in a state of health, each Element controls and moderates another Element in an appro-priate way. Water controls Fire, Fire controls Metal, Metal controls Wood, Wood controls Earth, and Earth controls Water. If this relationship breaks down and an Element becomes excessive or over-controlling, the cycle is no longer called the control cycle, but the "contempt cycle."

The commentator Zhang Jiebin underlines the situation where "heart and kidneys no longer communicate." When the heart has become weak and slack, timorous and clumsy, then fear and fright *kong ju* settle in and attack the power of the kidneys. The kidneys are now incapable of the control and containment that it is their duty to exercise; there is no longer firmness in their gathering and keeping.

Thus the symptoms of weight loss may be explained:

> The heart being depleted, the spleen is weak; this causes symptoms in well-developed forms and in the mass of flesh.
>
> *Zhang Jiebin*

At the joints where normally the accumulation of lubricants gives strength to the individual and to his movements, everything is flaccid, meager, and miserable. Where the abundance of flesh gives a healthy body its deliciously plump shape, there is now only emaciation and the disappearance of pleasant curves. The spleen, daughter of the heart and manifestation and formalization of expansion, is involved. The spleen is weakened by lack of nourishment from that which should enliven it − the Heart/Fire; and it is attacked by the organ/element that it should dominate − the Kidneys/Water. Caught between the perversion of Water and Fire, how could the Earth resist and survive? How could a clay pot that has not been fired have a shape that can resist soaking? Everything comes apart and is gone.

Naturally, the destruction of the corporeal form, emaciation, follows the loss of vitality, the loss (through leaking out) of the essences that should participate in the regeneration and maintenance of the flesh as well as in its nourishment.

Let us look for a moment at the expression *zi shi* 自失 (one loses possession of oneself). In a first approach it could be a loss *shi* 失 that comes from itself *zi* 自 , the simple consequence of the situation one has allowed to develop. Thus this loss could be a return to the condition where "there is a flowing out, there is a spilling over that cannot be stopped," as indicated by the first three statements in characters 227-292, lines 40-42.

The flowing out and spilling over that cannot be stopped by dikes or dams leads to the loss of the corporeal form by the attack on the flesh described in the reprise of these lines in lines 53-56.

But above all it is a question of the Spirits. Because the Spirits, and the guarding of the Spirits, guarantee self-possession, each one of us has a center, an inspired heart; each of us exists as a person, as an "I." But here there is flowing out and spilling over; we can no longer hold on to anything or contain ourselves. The essences are fleeing; the Spirits, vacillating under the emotional shock of apprehension and worry, are no longer guarded in their place and no longer guarantee the person. There is a dispossession of that which makes the person: one loses possession of oneself.

The expression for "one loses possession of oneself" *zi shi* is the inverse of another expression: to be in possession of, or take possession of, oneself *zi de* 自得. We see an example of this in the first chapter of the *Suwen* (cf. *The Way of Heaven*):

> Saints . . . on the outside do not encumber their bodies with business; inside themselves, they are not afflicted with worry *si xiang* 思想 ; they seek joyful serenity, putting all their concerns into the full possession of themselves *zi de*. An organism that is in a perfect state retains its essences and its Spirits *jing shen bu san* 精神不散 (the essences/Spirits do not disperse at all). Thus they can live one hundred years.

They (the Saints) did not die prematurely like those who allow themselves to be afflicted by worries and emotions of every kind.

The theme of premature death *yao* 夭 is taken up again (in characters 293-463), in each of the five stanzas (with the exception of the sixth) designating a *zang* attacked specifically by the emotions.

Signs of the internal undermining appear externally: the vegetation of the body – the body hair – becomes brittle; it is no longer nourished and irrigated, because the essences are impoverished or lost. The skin tone, the complexion *se* 色 , that should manifest the prospering of the blood and breaths and their good circulation, darkens, turns gray and pale, or it takes on whatever aspect would announce a premature death. Premature death does not mean dying young. It is dying from having wasted and misused one's vitality.

Balance and the presence of Spirits depends upon me, just as the "me," "I," exists only through them. The ills that touch me come from a blinding of the Spirits; they will finally cause premature death. Such a death was not in my original nature, in my heavenly endowment, or in my possibilities of flourishing.

Why have body hair and facial tone been singled out? Perhaps because together they constitute the visible body, because they are ruled by the heart and lung and give an account of the vitality of the whole (as do blood and breaths internally).

A person will die in the season where the aspect of movement that is attacked will fail most cruelly. Thus says Zhang Jiebin:

> When fire is diminished, one dreads water. Then there is death in winter.

In a more general way, the power of expansion and flourishing (the vital force that spreads out everywhere) being weakened by an attack upon the heart and its Spirits, one will die during the period where the opposite movement carries it off, where gathering and storing (the brake put on expansion) is most strongly manifested. In the vocabulary of the seasons, this is winter; it is also any moment in life, or in a situation, that has the same nature. Schematically this is explained in the cycle called the control or domination *ke* 克 cycle.

Nothing supports or makes up for the situation when winter comes; on the contrary, everything aggravates it: the external elements, the natural situations. So one dies of retraction and diminution, manifested in symptoms, as in our example, of weight loss.

When the Spleen falls prey to oppression and
*   sorrow and cannot free itself,*
The Intent is attacked.
When the Intent is attacked, one is disturbed until
*   the disorder is total,*
The four limbs can no longer rise.
The body hair becomes brittle and one has all the
*   signs of premature death.*
One dies in spring. (lines 59-64)

One can easily imagine how the Spleen, whose function is the harmonious distribution of breaths from a center and a turntable, can be deeply perturbed by an emotion that knots up the breaths and blocks their spreading.

Oppression *you* 憂 cannot be attributed easily to a particular *zang*: it is everything that prevents the development of a movement. Thus oppression occurs very often in relation to the lung; it has the same nature as the lung when the latter takes responsibility for gathering and squeezing, for the pressure that makes the liquids descend, and for the autumnal constraint. But in Chapter 5 of the *Suwen*, oppression also comes from the heart in reaction to a change. We also find oppression linked to the liver; it is the result of the essences/breaths' being annexed by the liver. Here the liver can no longer launch the forward movement of life, the starting-up movement is hampered, and the circulation of the breaths is knotted up. This is oppression *you*.

Thus, oppression attacks the lungs, and if it is too strong it prevents the lungs from propagating the breaths. But oppression can also attack other kinds of circulation: those that rule the liver, the heart, and the spleen. Here in *Lingshu* Chapter 8, it is the movements out from the spleen – permutation and distribution – that are attacked.

When the spleen is oppressed, how then can intent *yi* 意 be rooted and formed? How can it spread out with the breaths of the spleen and install order and harmony throughout the being? If intent, which is the spirit of the spleen, is absent or damaged, how can the permutations of different aspects of life be produced harmoniously? On the contrary, there can only be trouble and disorder. When intent collapses, the unfortunate state of the patient is described by two terms: bewilderment *men* 悗, and disorder *luan* 亂 . Nothing is more disconcerting than not knowing what one wants, nothing more distressing than disorder introduced into the activity of a person who has lost his concentration. Since it is the spleen that has responsibility for the barns and granaries, a responsibility that it shares with the stomach to assure the distribution of that which is essential for the maintenance of life, such bewilderment and disorder may cause serious problems.

As one no longer knows what to do and is incapable of correct movement, the problem shows up in the four limbs. They are no longer supported and nourished by supplies that depend on the spleen. Not only is strength lacking, but also the application of strength to activities is missing, because intent is absent. Conscious movements depend upon intent that is clear and capable of generating will.

Zhang Jiebin comments:

Oppression and sorrow *chou you* 愁憂: the breaths can no longer spread out with ease; the pathways of the network of animation *mai* 脉 are closed and obstructed. Oppression *you* is fundamentally a will *zhi* 志 linked to the lung; but it also attacks the spleen, because the breaths of mother and son communicate freely with one another. When there is oppression *you*, the breaths of the spleen are not at ease; there can no longer be transport and circulation *yun xing* 運行; thence disturbance and total disorder. The four limbs receive the breaths from the stomach, but only with the spleen's assistance. When the spleen is attacked, the four limbs are unable to rise.

One dies in springtime, the time of the year or the very moment in a situation where vitality should gush forth and impose itself everywhere with vivacity and swiftness. There is nothing to support this surge, and everything blocks and constrains it. *Yang*, freed into nature, presses upon the spleen, which is unable to follow the movement of spring (cf *The Way of Heaven*).

When the Liver falls prey to sadness and grief, one
is moved to one's center,
The Hun *are attacked, one loses reason and be*
comes forgetful; there is no vitality.
Without vitality one cannot guarantee the norm.
In this situation where the yin *apparatus contracts,*
where the musculature cramps,
The flanks on both sides can no longer rise.
The body hair becomes brittle and one has all the
signs of premature death.
One dies in autumn. (lines 65-72)

In several places in the *Neijing* the effects of sadness are described:

When there is sadness *bei* 悲 the breaths disappear. . . .
When there is sadness, the heart's connecting systems *xin xi* are constricted *ji* 急, the lung dilates and its leaves rise;[48] the

---

[48] This is the Chinese way of representing lungs, as if made up of leaves.

upper heater no longer guarantees its free communication; nutrition and defense *ying wei* 營衛 do not circulate; the breaths of heat are in the middle *zhong* 中 ; and in this way the breaths disappear.

Suwen, Chapter 39

Wang Bing recalls that the breaths of the lung are connected to all the meridians, the lung being master of the breaths, stimulating and giving rhythms to their circulations and disseminations. Thus when there is a counter-current the lung is dilated, and its "leaves" rise.

This is similar to Chapter 23 of the *Suwen*, which explains how sadness results from the lung's being taken over by the essences and breaths. This is the lung when it is attacked by sadness.

But sadness also touches the heart. Heart and lung form the upper heater, and that is why the upper heater no longer guarantees its free communication. The breaths cause obstructions that generate heat, making the breaths disappear, "devoured" by an excessive fire or heat. The breaths are melted, destroyed by heat (Fire prevailing over Metal in the *ke* cycle).

Sadness is the diametrical opposite of the joyful surge toward spreading out that is appropriate to the liver. *Bei* 悲、 (sadness) is a refusal. Through sadness we contradict our own desire to move ahead. Why are we so sad? Because we do not have a taste for the spontaneous effort that gives the vital movement.

The sadness *bei* that refuses life increases to a sadness that, by involution, fosters grief *ai* 哀 which can explode into groaning and shrieking from pain. The ensemble of sadness and grief *bei ai* 悲哀 constitutes a force, but one with inverted movement; instead of spreading its branches and its leaves in every direction, the springtime plant that I am turns against its own impetus, so now I attack my most inward self.

The effect is unmistakable. The *Hun – my Hun,* that part of me that accompanies the Spirits — no longer release like a mist that rises, but impeded in their release, they are panicked and forget themselves. *Kuang* 狂, madness and furious madness, is associated with *wang* 忘 , forgetfulness. We do not reproach the liver so much for its madness, as for the destruction of the personality. There is a healthy way of being mad and forgetful *kuang wang* 狂忘 : the lunacy of the mad monks whose "eccentricities" show how they are separate from the real lunacy of the worldly person whose life, while appearing well organized, is only a carefully maintained illusion.

Unfortunately there is a deadly madness, that of involution. By dint of going round and round, the individual cuts himself off from the necessary externalization, through lack of activity of his wounded *Hun*. An example of this cutting off is the schizophrenic, whose personality is already marked by depersonalization. Everyone has the right to be sad and aggrieved for a short while; but indulgence in these states postpones healing. There is a weakening of one's being, indicated by the text; no more vitality *jing* (essences): one can no longer replenish or strengthen one's essences.

The absence of essences in relation to the liver has the effect of upsetting the correctness of the way one leads one's life. In *Suwen* Chapter 8 (*Secret Treatise of the Spiritual Orchid*), the gall bladder is charged with assuring this correctness and rightness *zhong zhen* 中正 . Normality *zheng* 正 becomes aberration. The correct breaths *zheng* cannot release themselves from the deficient essences. The center *zhong* 中 is shaken; the norm no longer has a foundation. Some will say that the *shaoyang* fire, growing too strong, turns back on the Lung/Metal, drying up its *yin* fluids and destroying it (the contempt cycle).[49] This involution turns the life force against itself, rather than sending it outward.

Two passages from the *Neijing* (one from *Lingshu*, one from *Suwen*) assist our understanding of the preceding:

> When there is sadness and grief *bei ai*, and melancholy and chagrin *chou you*,[50] then the heart is moved *dong* 動 . When the heart is moved, then the Five *Zang* and the Six *Fu* are agitated; when they are agitated, the ancestral network of animation *zong mai* 宗脉[51] are affected (by suffering a pathogenic stimulation). When the *zong mai* are affected, the pathways of the dense liquids of the organism *ye dao* 液道 open, and since the pathways of the *ye* 液 are open, tears and mucus come out . . . (and as this loss of *ye* is a deprivation of the essences) the natural name is: deprived essences *duo jing*.
>
> *Lingshu*, Chapter 28

There is a clear relationship between sadness and grief and the flowing of tears; elsewhere these are all linked to the brain (i.e., cf *Suwen*,

---

[49] See Footnote 47.
[50] Oppression and sorrow.
[51] Power of unified command over the entire network of animation.

Chapter 81). Too great a loss of fluids through tears weakens the organism, the general equilibrium of the body and its *yin* riches, its treasure
of essences. We are deprived of our essences, of our vitality. *Lingshu*
Chapter 8 also asserts: one is without essences, without vitality. Further-
more, these essences normally guarantee the deep life of the brain and
the superior orifices. Therefore these upper regions are damaged by
sadness and grief.

> When sadness and grief *bei ai* are very intense, the net-
> work of liaisons of the innermost swaddlings (wrappings)
> *bao luo* 胞絡 is interrupted. When *bao luo* are interrupted,
> the *yang* breaths begin to move inside the interior *nei
> dong* 内動 . When this movement is unleashed, the heart
> makes things descend, as in hemorrhaging, and one fre-
> quently urinates blood.

Suwen, Chapter 44

Suwen Chapter 39 shows us how sadness prevents good circulation
in the upper heater and how, as a consequence, heat destroys the
breaths. We understand why the network of animation of the innermost swaddlings *bao luo* is interrupted and how the *yang* breaths are
excited. Blood leaves its vessels and even leaves the body, under the
pressure of the heat.

We can interpret *bao luo* as the path of liaisons linked to the uterus
(*bao* can designate the uterus or the innermost wrappings of the base
of the trunk), or as the network of wrapping and connections around
the heart (the *xin bao luo*); or even as an emanation from the *chongmai*
(*chong mo*).[52] In each case, there is an evil spreading of breaths, obstruction, and heat, provoking shakiness *dong* 動 in the interior. The heart's
defense and its communications are not assured. The kidneys are
implicated and the liver as well. The liver meridian is called the *jue yin*
of the foot, and the meridian corresponding to the *xin bao luo* is called
the *jue yin* of the hand. They are linked inside the *jue yin* quality of
the breaths. The liver stores the blood, and the *xin bao luo* helps the
circulation of the blood. If the blood is not following its path and the
communications with the heart are interrupted, how can the *Hun* be
illuminated by the heart Spirits, in order to conform to them and "follow
them faithfully?"

---

[52] One of the Eight Extraordinary Meridians.

When the *Hun* are no longer inspired and loss of blood diminishes the essences, the brain becomes weak (the liver meridian goes to the top of the head), and the essences no longer shine forth (cf *Suwen*, Chapter 17). Intelligence and clarity, depending upon the *Hun*, are attacked, giving rise to madness and forgetting *kuang wang* 狂忘.. This insanity is violent, because there is *yang* agitation and heat.

The musculature system is normally centered upon the *yin* genital apparatus and its dependencies (cf. *zong jin* 宗筋 , "the ancestral muscle," the command post for the muscular strength of the entire body); it expands and contracts. Here the pathology is that it retracts and turns inward, rather than moving outward.

Normally the general muscular activity is also deployed peripherally. When pathological, this periphery knots up and cramps. Knotting up is the periphal aspect of pathology here, and retracting is its central aspect.

Pursuing the description of muscular atony, we complete what has been said about the pathology of the center and of the periphery by indicating the pathology along the axillaries, in the area of the ribs. Immobilization of the bones beneath the axillaries is a consequence of the retraction of the *yin* apparatus and of the cramping of the musculature. The symptoms are located along the pathways of animation of the liver.

Death comes in autumn, the season when *yang* gives way to *yin*. The discomfort already present is doubled by the effects of the *yin* ambience brought by autumn. One dies in autumn, or at any period that has the qualities or nature of autumn. One dies when everything is being gathered in; there is no more spreading out or blossoming. One dies at the harvest of the breaths (for here the breaths are annihilated) and of the Spirits (for they are no longer guarded by the essences which are deficient, nor by the *Hun* which are under attack).

When the Lung falls prey to boundless elation and joy,
The Po *are attacked.*
When the Po *are attacked, one loses reason.*
With this loss of reason, the Intent knows no one,
The skin shrivels and wrinkles.

The body hair becomes brittle and one has all the
signs of premature death.
One dies in summer. (lines 73-79)

Why do we reproach elation and joy? Because they have no boundaries *wu ji* 無極. They are whipped up by the desire to be always more and more and more. If nothing opposes this, it develops everywhere, uncontrollably. It is an excitement that causes the fulcrum of life and of the Spirits to leap and gush out. The foundations, aroused by elation and joy, are carried away by unbridled movement towards the exterior.

The *Po*, whose service is strictly defined and tied to the essences, are washed away and carried far off from their tasks. Nothing is as it should be. The bolting *yang* attack the *Po* which are associated with the essences. The natural and instinctive conduct of life is perverted; the normal conduct of the human being becomes aberrant.

The *Po* go mad in their own way, and we speak of *kuang* 狂 (madness, violent lunacy, wildness), as we do when the *Hun* go crazy in their own way. But we do not say that the *Po* are forgetful *wang* 忘; that identity crisis pertains to the *Hun* which are higher authorities. The crisis of the *Po* points out the difference between *Hun* and *Po*.

The attacked *Po* transmit to the intent *yi* 意 the blow they have received. The intent, shaken, accentuates the state of madness. Whatever is without purpose cannot last *bu cun* 不存 in an individual. The intimate connection capable of maintaining vital movement no longer exists. No longer do the corporeal souls implement the spiritual souls, inverting the proposition made by Laozi in Chapter 10:

> In bringing your spiritual souls together with the physical
> ones, embracing Unity, can you keep them together?

The same character *kuang* is used to express madness in the case of the attack upon the *Hun*, as in that upon the *Po* (In the latter, it is madness that follows an excess of *yang*.). When the liver fell prey to sadness and grief, the *yang* power turned against the internal vitality and brought on death through retraction, a pulling in. When the lung falls prey to elation and joy, the *yang* power pulls everything to the outside, bringing on death because one's life is ablaze, burning at every extremity.

The heart, weakened by the spilling out of its appropriate feelings of elation and joy, is incapable of correctly generating the spleen, and one cannot conserve one's intent.[53] When the weakened heart can no longer apply itself, how can authentic intent come into being? When intent cannot persevere, there is no possibility of real will *zhi*, nor of a sound and sensible orientation of the mind and emotions. Neither thought nor reflection can form correctly.

When intent is incapable of being a matrix for will and thought, or of recognizing and considering things and beings, there is unrestrained behavior, where human relations are ridiculed (by the afflicted person), and the relationships between the innermost part and the exterior are derailed. Intent becomes ignorant of others *yi bu cun ren* 意不存人; there is no perseverance of intent; it is the end of the relations which make a man.

At this point, the heart Fire is too strong, and it invades the Metal of the lung (*ke* cycle of domination); this propels the breaths from the lung in every direction. Full of perverse heat, they blow out all the way to the skin, which is in communion with the lung; then the skin shows symptoms of shriveling and wrinkling. In addition, Fire's attack on Metal also provokes an attack on the *Po* with these consequences, according to Zhang Jiebin:

> Elation gushes out of the heart; joy spreads to the exterior. Violent elations attack the *yang*; this is why the Spirits/breaths *shen qi* are scared away and dispersed and no longer stored in place. To be scared away is to be filled with fear and the movement of fright.
>
> Elation finds its root in the heart's will *zhi*, and it attacks the lung. Violent elations attack the *yang*; the perversities of Fire straddle the Metal. When the *Po* are attacked, the Spirits are in disarray and this causes loss of reason, or madness *kuang*. Intent is not conserved in man. He ignores others *yi bu cun ren* 意不存人, as if there were no one nearby. The skin is the union *he* 合 of the lung.

---

[53] This is the perspective of Ma Shi.

One dies in summer, when the external heat and the natural disposition of the season towards externalization encourage the perverse
tendency and deliver the final blow to the depletion of essences within.

When the Kidneys fall prey to anger that swells
without stopping,
The Will is attacked, one can no longer even remem-
ber what one has just said,
The loins and dorsal spine can neither lean forward
nor lean backward,
Neither bend, nor straighten.
The body hair becomes brittle and one has all the
signs of premature death.
One dies in the last stage of summer. (lines 80-85)

Violent anger takes everything up in a counter-current that empties the
lower part. Breaths and blood rush up, pressure is exerted transversely
towards the organs located in the path of this counter-current: those of
the middle and upper heaters. This explains the faculty of forgetting *xi
wang* 喜忘 or, according to a different reading of the text, elation *xi*
accompanied by memory loss *wang* 忘, pertaining to "what one has just
said." This means awareness is limited to the very moment that a person
is speaking or being.

The kidneys are carried away by swelling anger without anyone's
being able to stop them, or without their being able to stop themselves.
The attack upon the special authority of the kidneys — the will *zhi* —
produces a disruption of the personality.

To be a man, one must remember the man one has been. This man
who once was exists totally in the "what one has just said" *qian yan* 前言 [54]
The literal meaning of these words (to retain in one's memory what one
has just said) is not unimportant, but above all one must keep or conserve
the quality of the man who expresses himself through what he says. The
word comes from the heart; the complete expression of oneself lies in
one's word *xin* 信, [55] (confidence, assurance). How could we have con-

---

[54] "The words pronounced before," the words one has pronounced in the previous
moment.
[55] Man 亻 and word 言

fidence in one who has already lost for himself the creative rapport of the personality that unites man 人 to his expression 言 ? The value of this short declaration lies in reminding us that each person's objectivity rests upon the soundness of his subjectivity.

This is all a matter of the will *zhi* held in the kidneys. Beware of exaggeration *sheng* 盛 , which gives the appearance of strength, but which in reality is weakness turned toward oneself. Beware also of anger *nu* 怒 with the appearance of violent terror, which in reality is an aberration turned usually toward others.

Swelled anger *sheng nu* 盛怒 is a trap. It is carried away by itself in the same way, and for the same reasons (as we have seen) that elation is enraptured by itself and also carried away. Joy always wants to increase more and more. The vocabulary used in discussing the difference between the lung's and the kidneys' expansive nature is interesting to note. The lung's business is to spread out into the immensity of space; thus what disturbs it tends to fill the cosmos like an expanding gas. The kidneys' business is the outpouring of the hidden source of life that flows and wants to flow indefinitely without exhausting itself unduly. In the first case, the lung's exaltation is said to be "without boundaries" *wu ji* 無極; it wants to be limitless. In the case of the kidneys, their exaltation is said to be "without stopping" *bu zhi* 不止 ; it (the exaltation) knows no cessation; it wants to flow forever.

The effects of weakened kidneys go to the bones, especially to the eminent command post in the lumbar region and, beyond, to the entire vertebral column (cf *Suwen* Chapter 3). Movement is no longer possible; there is no longer any suppleness. This goes well with the idea we have of anger, which is said to stiffen rather than soften, to immobilize in position and not turn and move about.

The will makes a being move without stiffness; it promotes the flexibility of all attitudes and sustains thought without rigidity. The will is the deep power, the structuring of the mind, which has its physical expression in the bones, particularly in those that provide the structure from the base of the trunk to the head. Anger, emptying the base, attacks the will as well as the bones, through causing the deterioration of the essences. The structure, whether it be the will or the bones, is the opposite of rigidity; it is efficient suppleness, strong and sure movement, like that of a gymnast.

The continuity of a being is damaged by an attack on the will and the bones, and by the above-mentioned loss of memory of what has just been said. One can no longer maintain a will, a tendency, or a general and coherent tension of the vital movement.

Orderly control of life thus becomes impossible in such a situation.

> Anger—the breaths are going in a counter-current *nu*; when it intensifies, there is necessarily disorder *luan* 亂 ; from this comes disturbance and uncontrollable *bu zhi* aberration.
>
> Anger is fundamentally a will of the liver; but it also attacks the kidneys, because liver and kidneys are son and mother, and their breaths are in mutual communication. When the will *zhi* is attacked, then intent *yi* is lost; this results in forgetting what one has just said.
>
> The lumbar region *yao* 腰 is the storehouse *fu* 府 of the kidneys.
>
> *Zhang Jiebin*

One dies in the last stages of summer; water in decline fears the victorious earth. The fire of anger, pushing up, can only double the difficulties of the moment of passing from the *yang* seasons to the *yin* seasons, of the moment when the current is reversed to return to the depths, where its vivacity will be reduced and controlled.

*Under the effect of fear and fright from which one
  cannot free oneself,
The Essences are attacked, the bones grow stiff,
  impotence leads to withdrawal.
At times the Essences descend by themselves. (lines 86-88)*

The five preceding groupings of lines show the attack upon the essences through the seizure of each of the five *zang* by an emotion. Now we have a sixth group, recapitulating and concluding lines 53-88. It is a presentation of direct attack upon the essences themselves.

> With fear and dread the Spirits are frightened, and they disperse. . . . Heart and kidneys receive the attack.
>
> In the case of fear, the breaths descend and collapse; this is why the essences are attacked. The kidneys master the

bones; thus, when the essences are attacked, the bones grow stiff. The impotence *wei* 痿 in question is sexual impotence *yang wei* 陽痿, and the withdrawal *jue* 厥 is the decline of *yang*.

Ming men 命門 does not guard *bu shou* 不守 (is not guarded), so the essences at times descend by themselves; the storing ability (thesaurization) of the kidneys has taken the attack.

Zhang Jiebin

Zhang Zhicong reminds us:

The essences of Fire make the Spirits; the essences of Water make the will *zhi*. We have spoken of *Hun*, *Po*, will, intent; all of those are rooted in the essences/Spirits *jing shen* of heart and kidneys in order to be produced *sheng* 生 [56]. This is why apprehension and anxiety, worry and preoccupation attack the Spirits. But we have not yet spoken of fear and fright *kong ju* 恐懼 without the possibility of freeing ourselves from that which attacks the essences. The Spirits are born of the essences, and the essences turn back *gui* 歸 to the Spirits.

There is no clearer way to say that the heart and kidneys are attacked; that fear and fright have so shaken the foundations of the being that the solidity of life, and of the primary essences, is lost from the place where they have been stored and have been active since the beginning. This place, after the time of the *Neijing*, will be called *mingmen*; it is the other face of the kidneys.

The beginning of *Lingshu* Chapter 8 shows us the Spirits springing forth from the double essences.[57] This means that throughout the life of a being, Spirits continually appear out of one's essences, and through one's essences. This is *jing shen*, epitomizing the activity of the five *zang*, under the authority of the heart and the kidneys.

If the attack goes all the way to the original essences, the vitality is shaken to the innermost depths: the bones in their interior and in their strength, not simply in their motor capacity and their flexibility and suppleness. The strength of the kidneys and of the original essences is expressed by the strength of the bones, as well as by the strength of

---

[56] Vitalized
[57] See line 21 (at characters 84-186). Double essences mean the essences of Heaven and Earth becoming Virtue and Breaths within a being, expressed as *yin/yang*.

one's reproductive power. Hence the possibility of two interpretations for the character *wei* 痿 , impotence: it can relate to the bones or to sexual strength, and sometimes to both. The polymorphic attack falls on one's power. Power is linked to the kidneys and to the original essences. Whether one becomes impotent, paralyzed, numb, weak, or powerless, it is a variation of the expression of loss of power.

If the attack is on the original essences, the original Fire is weakened. Being unable to spread out anywhere, the decrease of *yang* will drag along withdrawal *jue* 厥 .[58] Emptiness caused by the absence or lack of something allows the perverse to intrude.

This is not the first time in the *Neijing* that we see a series of six propositions, of which the first five refer to the five *zang* and the last to the origin, expressed through rapport with the kidneys as conservators of the origin, and with the essences as original realities.

In the last instance, there is no particular season for death: it is the loss of *yang*, of life, through loss of *yin* and of the essences. Death arises from the interior of a being, and not through gross failure to adapt to external circumstances.

The condition of the essences descending by themselves is much worse than spermatorrhea. This is because there is a deviation from the correct movement of the essences, which should take them to meet the Spirits in the great relationship between kidneys and heart. The essences have lost their identity and no longer fulfill their role: thus there is deep weakening of the bones, and the loss or flowing out that we have already seen (in lines 42-44 of characters 227-292) as a consequence of fear and fright. Thus the first attack was upon the Spirits, under the effect of apprehension and anxiety, of worry and preoccupation. Here, the essences are attacked directly. The solidarity of the essences and the Spirits is involved; what disintegrates is the *jing shen* (essences/Spirits), which are at once the expression and manifestation of the individual life at its highest level, the compenetration of Water and Fire, the meeting of above and below, and the model of a perfect, essential, and inspired relationship.

---

[58] *Jue* is a lack of strength in the distribution of essences/breaths so that they no longer reach the totality of the regions that they should occupy, creating lack and voids. Perversion will then take advantage of the voids to intrude.

This is why the Five *Zang*, whose function is to master and
    to store the Essences,
Must not be attacked at all.   90
For if they suffer attacks, their guard is no longer upheld,
And the *yin* becomes empty.
Empty *yin* is the absence of Breaths,
And the absence of Breaths is, quite simply, death.

This being so, one who wishes to use needles   95
Must examine attentively the way the ill person presents
    himself,
To perceive the preservation or the disappearance of the
    Essences and Spirits, the *Hun* and the *Po*,
And whether the inner disposition is favorable or
    unfavorable.

If those five are attacked, the needle cannot treat.

Characters 464 to 527

是故五臟主藏精者也
shi gu wu zang zhu cang jing zhe ye

不可傷
bu ke shang

傷則失守而陰虛
shang ze shi shou er yin xu

陰虛則無氣
yin xu ze wu qi

無氣則死矣
wu qi ze si yi

是故用針者
shi gu yong zhen zhe

察觀病人之態
cha guan bing ren zhi tai

以知精神魂魄之存亡
yi zhi jing shen hun po zhi cun wang

得失之意
de shi zhi yi

五者以傷針不可以治之也
wu zhe yi shang zhen bu ke yi zhi zhi ye

This is why the Five Zang, *whose function is to*
   master and to store the Essences,
Must not be attacked at all.
For if they suffer attacks, their guard is no longer
   upheld,
And the yin *becomes empty.*
Empty yin *is the absence of Breaths,*
And the absence of Breaths is, quite simply, death.
   (lines 89-94)

The first part of the text ("This is why the five *zang* . . . is, quite simply, death.") is a conclusion.

> This is a resume of all the preceding. The five *zang* each have their essences, and if they suffer an attack, then the *yin* empties, for the essences of the five *zang* are the *yin*. When the *yin* is empty, there are no longer any breaths, for it is through the essences that the breaths may appear over the course of transformations. When the breaths accumulate, there is life; when the breaths dissipate, there is death. Thus, death and life are in the breaths, and the breaths are rooted in the essences.
>
> *Zhang Jiebin*

But let us not forget that beyond the breaths, the guarding of the *zang* bears on the Spirits and on the particular Spirit of each *zang*. The *Taisu* is more sensitive to this aspect:

> The Spirits *shen* 神 of the five *zang* cannot take an attack. If the five *shen* are attacked, the *shen* leave and there is no longer any guard; the storing and the guarding are lost. . . .
> The *Dao* for not dying is to nourish, *yang* 養 , the five spirits *wu shen* 五神 .

Maintaining the Five Spirits means maintaining the individual Spirits of each of the Five *zang* in their own specificity and harmony within the whole. The primary condition of this is impregnation and saturation of the *zang* by quality essences.

There seems no reason to differentiate between the essences of Anterior Heaven and those of Posterior Heaven. The harmonious conjunction of both within the individual permits the releasing of the breaths, the enlivening presence of the Spirits, and finally, the accomplishment of one's natural life span.

The essences stored by the Five *Zang* must not receive the attack, since they are the basis of vitality and of its reconstitution, the foundation of a being's structure, and the guarantee of protection for the Spirits. The essences are the *yin*. The *yang* is rooted in the *yin*. The essences are the starting point for the "transformations of the breaths," the releasing and production of breaths through transformations of the essences. Thus, when the *yin* empties, there are no more breaths. The breaths are the strength of the movements of life. When the breaths are gone, life ceases; there is death.

This being so, one who wishes to use needles
Must examine attentively the way the ill person
    presents himself,
To perceive the preservation or the disappearance
    of the Essences and Spirits, the **Hun** *and the* **Po***,*
And whether the inner disposition is favorable or
    unfavorable.

If those five are attacked, the needle cannot treat.
    (lines 95-99)

The second part of the text (". . . one who wishes to use needles . . . the needle cannot treat.") deals with applying the previously stated doctrine to therapeutic practice, to the manipulation of needles.

If one perceives that the patient is unable, in his internal alchemy, to let life express itself and to direct his Spirits, it is useless to place the needles. If the intimate thesaurization of the essences has been gravely hit, one places the needle in vain. It is like trying to slice water with a sword.

A true internal deficiency – an emptiness of *yin* – cannot be treated by needles. Such a treatment requires that the breaths of the patient collaborate. If this is lacking, one will try to rebuild the *yin* through the use of drugs and diverse medications. Zhang Jiebin's position:

> When needles are used, all one can do is consider the aspect presented by the ill person, in order to decide whether or not one can utilize the needle. When the essences/Spirits *jing shen* of the Five *Zang* are deteriorated and damaged, one must not dream of using needles.

Chapter 37 of *Lingshu* says: "When blood and breaths are overabundant, the flesh is full and firm and can tolerate the needles."

Chapter 4 of *Lingshu* says: "If all (the *mai*, the pulses) are small, *yin* and *yang*, body and breaths, are insufficient; in this case do not use needles, but instead use sweet drugs *gan yao* 甘藥 to regulate *tiao* 調 ."

Chapter 5 of *Lingshu* says: "When body and breaths are insufficient, the breaths of the ill person are insufficient; the *yin* as well as *yang* breaths are insufficient; one cannot place a needle."

From all of that, we see clearly that needles have the capacity to treat overabundance, but cannot treat emptiness and deterioration. Thus one must be very careful with needle manipulation.

Being careful with needle manipulation means not taking their use lightly. But to determine truly whether needles can be used or not, one must go all the way to an examination of the Spirits, as the rooting in the Spirits is the subject of *Lingshu* Chapter 8.

It is not yet a question of deciding between the use of needles or that of medicaments, of distinguishing between overabundance and insufficiency. One must first go to the root, to find out how the patient's Spirits are.

If we look carefully at the text, we see that it speaks of the intent *yi* that is perceived in the patient: we must know if this intent is in a state of acquisition/ possession *de* 得 , or of loss *shi* 失 : whether one is in possession of oneself or in the process of losing one's life. Possession implies the possibility of taking hold of oneself again; loss implies the inexorable flight of a life that is escaping, because it neither belongs any longer, nor does it have any way to want to return again. This refers to the inner disposition of the patient, favorable or unfavorable.

Before examining the intent *yi*, however, it is necessary to perceive the maintenance or the disappearance of essences and Spirits, of the *Hun* and *Po*. This is the order of presentation of the first four authorities (lines 21-24, at characters 84-186), coming immediately after the appearance of life *sheng* 生 given at the beginning of *Lingshu* Chapter 8. It is their fertile embrace that makes and maintains life; if they untie themselves and come apart, death is near, and without remedy.

Let us look at the stylistic arrangement of the statement. We notice five succeeding terms. They are: Essences, Spirits, *Hun*, *Po*, and – slightly detached – Intent *yi*, which is given special treatment.

Essences, Spirits, *Hun* and *Po* were presented before the Heart (lines 21-24). Those four end, so to speak, at the arrival of the Heart. Intent, however, comes out of the Heart and is the first authority to do so. The authorities that culminate in Knowing-how (the knowledge necessary for maintenance of life) come from the transformation of Intent. This difference explains the special treatment given to Intent. Essences, Spirits, *Hun* and *Po* are the superior emanations that fasten life within us. They remain, holding us and holding on to us, or they are at the point of unfastening, dissolving and destroying us. Intent is the first expression of our own life, responsible, fully assumed, capable of governing the orientation that depends on us: it is turned toward acquisition/possession or loss, the *de shi* 得失, that sums up all of existence.

The therapist must perceive the condition of the Essences, Spirits, *Hun*, *Po*, and Intent. If the essences and the Spirits, the *Hun* and the *Po* are at the point of unfastening and separating, if Intent is not oriented in such a way that it can generate a strong Will and retain the Spirits which are in the process of divorce, then nothing – neither needles, nor medicines – will make any difference. The being is already lost, has lost himself. Internally the five *zang* have been struck, the spirits of the five *zang* are under attack, and they are going to leave.

> The essential point in the treatment of an illness is to root oneself in the five Spirits of the person: to know whether they dwell or have been lost, whether one possesses or loses them (whether one is in a state of possession or of loss), to know if the intent *yi* is for death or for life. And then one prescribes needles and medications to circulate, harmonize, and maintain.
>
> If, following debauchery and excess *zong yi* 縱逸, the five Spirits are attacked, and if the physician does not inform himself of the dwelling or the loss of the Spirits/breaths *shen qi*, and even worse, if he treats by using needles and medicaments, one will inevitably end in premature death.
>
> *Taisu*

According to this severe commentary of *Taisu*, all treatment will only hasten death, by further weakening the ill person, using up his strength in vain efforts or in desperate resistance.

The Liver stores the Blood, the Blood is the dwelling place
of the *Hun*. 100
When the Breaths of the Liver are empty, there is fear.
When they are full, there is anger.

The Spleen stores the *ying*; the *ying* is the dwelling place
of Intent.
When the breaths of the Spleen are empty, the four limbs
can no longer be of any use,
And the Five *Zang* know no peace. 105
Whey they are full, the belly is swollen, transits and
micturition function badly.

The Heart stores the *mai*; the *mai* are the dwelling place of
the Spirits.
When the breaths of the Heart are empty, there is sadness.
When they are full, one laughs without being able to stop.

The Lung stores the Breaths; the Breaths are the
dwelling place of the *Po*. 110
When the Breaths of the Lung are empty, the nose is
stopped up and functions poorly;
The Breaths diminish.
When they are full, one gasps noisily; the chest is
constricted;
One must raise the head to breathe.

The Kidneys store the Essences; the Essences are the
dwelling place of the Will. 115
When the breaths of the Kidneys are empty, there is
withdrawal.
When they are full, there is swelling, and the Five *Zang*
know no peace.

Characters 528 to 644

肝 藏 血 血 舍 魂
gan cang xue xue she hun

肝 氣 虛 則 恐
gan qi xu ze kong

實 則 怒
shi ze nu

脾 藏 營 營 舍 意
pi cang ying ying she yi

脾 氣 虛 則 四 肢 不 用
pi qi xu ze si zhi bu yong

五 臟 不 安
wu zang bu an

實 則 腹 脹 經 溲 不 利
shi ze fu zhang jing sou bu li

心 藏 脈 脈 舍 神
xin cang mai mai she shen

心 氣 虛 則 悲
xin qi xu ze bei

實 則 笑 不 休
shi ze xiao bu xiu

肺 藏 氣 氣 舍 魄
fei cang qi qi she po

肺 氣 虛 則 鼻 塞 不 利 少 氣
fei qi xu ze bi se bu li shao qi

實 則 喘 喝 胸 盈 仰 息
shi ze chuan he xiong ying yang xi

腎 藏 精 精 舍 志
shen cang jing jing she zhi

腎 氣 虛 則 厥
shen qi xu ze jue

實 則 脹 五 臟 不 安
shi ze zhang wu zang bu an

It will be necessary to discern with care the symptoms of
pathology of the Five *Zang*,

In order to be in a position to perceive the emptiness or
fullness of their breaths.

120

Be aware of this when you treat someone.

Characters 528 to 644 (cont.)

必 審 五 臟 之 病 形
bi shen wu zang zhi bing xing

以 知 其 氣 之 虛 實
yi zhi qi qi zhi xu shi

謹 而 調 之 也
jin er tiao zhi ye

We have seen that the feelings can activate, internally, the process leading to death. Now we must determine via what external clinical signs and via what sorts of superficial manifestations of interior conditions the therapist will grasp the *zang* whose spirits are disturbed. In addition, one must distinguish two possible cases: emptiness or fullness.

> Liver, heart, spleen, lung and kidneys are called the Five
> *Zang, wu zang* 五臟 (the five which store, thesaurize); they
> thesaurize *cang* 藏 the essences/breaths *jing qi* 精氣.
> Blood *xue*, the network of animation *mai*, deep nutritive
> reconstruction *ying* 營 , breaths *qi*, and essences *jing* are
> called the five essences/breaths *wu jing qi* 五精氣; they house
> *she* 舍 the five Spirits *wu shen* 五神.
>
> *Taisu*

The function of each organ *zang* is to actively store the essences in its own proper way, in order to release from those essences the breaths that are specific to the moment of over-all animation of the Being whose *zang* it is. The different specific emanations that manifest within us in the activity of each *zang* are called essences/breaths *jing qi*. The influence of the Spirits is propagated through these emanations. The Spirits also are known by the activity of each *zang* and recognized by the characteristics appropriate to each one. Thus blood, *mai*, nutrition, breaths, and essences are the dwelling places of the *Hun*, the *Shen*, Intent, the *Po*, and the Will — the five Spirits.

The unity of the *Shen* Spirits is unbroken; it differentiates and takes form through the activities of the *zang*, which are the five polarities, or moments of animation. The Heart, whose central and dominant position has been shown, takes the *Shen* for its own Spirits. The other *zang* manifest their own Spirits in *Hun*, *Po*, Intent, and Will. This ensemble is called "the Five Spirits" *wu shen*. Another name for it is "that which the Five *Zang* store" *wu zang suo cang* 五臟所藏, as in the *Suwen*, Chapter 23.

> The breaths of the Five *Zang* each have their emptiness
> and fullness, and one can distinguish their differences through
> diagnosis. The Five *Zang* each have that which they store,
> and the five wills *wu zhi* 五志 each have a place to dwell.
> If the five wills receive a blow, there are illnesses of the five
> wills. If the breaths of the *zang* are not balanced, symptoms
> of the breaths of the *zang* appear. This is why one must

observe the aspects that the illnesses of the five *zang* show, in order to know the deficiency or the excessiveness of their breaths.

Zhang Zhicong

If a *zang* is incapable of sustaining the tendency and the tension of life for which it is responsible, or if its strength tangles and overflows, specific symptoms can be read, and from them one can deduce the condition of the entire mind or – to conform to traditional expression – of the Spirits of a subject.

The Liver stores the Blood; the Blood is the dwelling place of the Hun.
When the Breaths of the Liver are empty, there is fear.
When they are full, there is anger. *(lines 100-102)*

The connection between Liver, Blood and *Hun* are pointed out several times in the *Neijing*:

> The Liver stores the *Hun*.
>
> *Suwen*, Chapter 23

> When man is at rest, the blood returns to the liver.
>
> *Suwen*, Chapter 10

> The liver stores the blood. . . . When there is an overabundance of blood, there is 'anger. . . . When there is insufficiency, there is fear.
>
> *Suwen*, Chapter 62

We also remember the *Suwen*, Chapter 8 (cf *Secret Treatise of the Spiritual Orchid*), where the liver is given the charge of being General of the Army, who must beware of both fear and rage.

In *Cascade I* we have presented a study of the *Hun* and their relationship with the blood. Let us add simply that the liver expands its power thanks to the arrival of fresh troops represented by the blood; that the sanguine liquid is co-penetrated by the airy and subtle emanations of the *Hun*; that the two express the duality of the liver that is rooted in the *yin* (in the Water of the kidneys) and shows the effects of its *yang* power in its function of thrust and projection. In addition, by means of the blood whose circulation is obedient to the heart, the *Hun* can effectively "follow the Spirits faithfully."

We understand that the abundant sanguine mass, subjected to an excess power of the breaths of the liver, can be enlivened to a rising and a raging that, at the level of feelings, is anger; and conversely, a weakness of these breaths engenders a slackening and letting go, a downward movement. This weakness and sinking is the nature of fear.

> The liver has mastery over the musculature; when the time is right for a man to rest, the blood returns to the liver; this is how the *Hun* are able to dwell in the blood. The kidneys store the water; the liver stores the wood and masters anger. Water engenders wood, and when the liver (the son) is empty the kidneys (the mother) overlap it, and thus with emptiness of the liver there is fear.
>
> *Taisu*

The *Taisu* explains the pathologies described in this fragment in terms of the mother-son relationship (with the exception of spleen and lung, the two *tai yin*). It also adopts an order of presentation that differs slightly from the usual editions of *Lingshu*. This order is the begetting *sheng* cycle, in which the liver begets the heart, the heart begets the spleen, the spleen begets the lung, the lung begets the kidney, and the kidney begets the liver. The *Taisu*'s commentary should not be allowed to overshadow the movement of life that is deeper than what is only touched upon by the mother-son rule, nor all the relationships that are the very mark of life both in its normality and in its disturbance.

The Spleen stores the ying; *the* ying *is the dwelling place of Intent.*
When the breaths of the Spleen are empty, the four limbs can no longer be of any use,
And the Five Zang *know no peace.*
When they are full, the belly is swollen, transits and micturition function badly. (lines 103-106)

> The Spleen thesaurizes Intent.
>
> *Suwen*, Chapter 23

The spleen thesaurizes the flesh *rou* 肉 .... In an over-abundance of the corporeal form *xing* 形, the belly is swollen, and transit and micturition function poorly. In insufficiency, the four limbs are no longer able to be of any use.

Suwen, Chapter 62

Intent presents form; it formalizes. *Ying* 營 offers maintenance and reconstruction; it renews the forms of the body. The natural movement of the spleen is expressed this way. The whole being, from the most external (as in the four limbs) to the most internal (as in the five *zang*), depends upon this nutritive maintenance, this permanent remodeling. Thought and activities of the consciousness depend on the nutrition that comes from the spleen, "the barns and granaries" of the being. When the spleen cannot correctly send out, maintain, and renew vitality, the four limbs are weakened. It can be said that the intent has also become impotent and no longer guides the movements of the limbs which, reciprocally, are incapable of following the incitements of intent and the will. More profoundly, the five *zang* lose their alimentation, and their essences are incapable of a harmonious synergy. The battle is on for whatever portion is available; there is weakness and disorder. The Five *Zang* are not peaceful.

In the case of fullness, despite an abundance that can hardly be assimilated, there is blockage and congestion instead of enrichment. The belly is the chosen site of the congestions of the spleen's excess breaths. The bottleneck blocks circulations, including circulations moving towards the outside of the body. It seems that the two terms used, *jing sou* 經溲, designate together the possible passages: the two needs (the two routes of evacuation: urination and defecation), and also the woman's menses.

> *Ying* is the blood and the flesh.
> The spleen rules the liquids and cereals (grains); it is master of the *zang* and *fu*. When it is empty, the four limbs (that depend on the *fu*, which are yang) are useless, and the *zang*, which are *yin*, have no peace. When there is fullness, there is swelling and blockage that can affect the woman's menses as well as the large and the small need.
>
> *Taisu*

The *ying* comes out at the middle heater; it receives the breaths, it seizes the juices; through change and transformations it becomes red, and that indicates blood. This is why it is said that the spleen stores the *ying*. The *ying* is the home of intent *yi*; the spleen stores intent.

When the spleen is empty, the four limbs are useless and the five *zang* have no peace; this is because the spleen rules the four limbs, and because the spleen is the origin *yuan* of the five *zang* (i.e., the source of their renewal).

The *mai* of the *taiyin* penetrate the belly and have a relationship of connection *luo* 絡 with the stomach; this is why, when the spleen is full, the belly is swollen, and transits and micturition function poorly.

Zhang Jiebin

The Heart stores the mai; the mai are the dwelling place of the Spirits.
When the breaths of the Heart are empty, there is sadness.
When they are full, one laughs without being able to stop. (lines 107-109)

> The Heart stores the *Shen*. . . . The Heart masters the *mai*.
>
> Suwen, Chapter 23

> The heart stores the *Shen*. . . . When the Spirits *shen* are overabundant, one laughs uncontrollably. . . . When the Spirits are insufficient, one is sad.
>
> Suwen, Chapter 62

By its mastery of the entire network of animation (the *mai*), and especially of the way the *mai* assures the circulation of the blood *xue mai*, the heart propagates life and the radiance of the Spirits everywhere. The superior activities — those headquartered in and commanded by the heart[59] — inform and re-make each fragment of the being. The happiness of being alive is manifested everywhere.

---

[59] Under obedience to the heart as conceived by Ancient China.

Pathological emptiness thus shows as a sadness *bei* that is a refusal of joy, causing one to mourn life within oneself. Fullness shows as an excitation that is externalized without limit and without ceasing. A smile is appropriate to the joy of the heart, but the intemperate and immoderate manifestation of wild laughter is not.

> The liver stores the wood; it masters sadness and grief *bei ai* 悲哀. The heart stores the fire; it masters laughter. Wood begets fire; thus when the son, the heart, is (pathologically) empty, the mother, the liver, overlaps. So there is sadness when the heart is empty.
>
> *Taisu*

This explanation of the *Taisu* seems a bit systematic. It is more satisfactory to consider the aspect of the vital movement that the heart represents: the expansion and deployment manifested by the network of animation (the *mai*) and exemplified by the Spirits at the highest level. Among the feelings, joy of life is the normal expression felt. Weakened, it is sadness; exaggerated, it is laughter; either one is a loss of control by the Spirits, by the heart.

**The Lung stores the Breaths; the Breaths are the
   dwelling place of the Po.
When the Breaths of the Lung are empty, the nose is
   stopped up and functions poorly;
The Breaths diminish.
When they are full, one gasps noisily; the chest is
   constricted;
One must raise the head to breathe.** *(lines 110-114)*

> The Lung stores the *Po*.
>
> *Suwen*, Chapter 23

> The lung stores the breaths. . . . When there is overabundance of breaths, there is gasping and coughing, a rising of the breaths. When there is insufficiency, respiration is scarce and the breaths are diminished.
>
> *Suwen*, Chapter 62

The lung rules the breaths of the entire body; it propagates them within the organism and gives rhythm to their distribution; it commands respiration. The breaths of the lung give to the *Po* (which are of the same nature as the essences) the strength and the dynamism they need. When the breaths of the lung are weak, the *Po* lack strength also.

The breaths of respiration enter via the nose. When the lung is weak, the perverse breaths will easily penetrate there and settle in. The nose is stopped up; breathing becomes weak and incapable of propagating the breaths as usual. These breaths dwindle and diminish.

When there is fullness, the area of the chest and diaphragm is blocked. The passages are constricted (as they were with the spleen at a lower level); breathing is painful and noisy. . . . One must raise the head to find breath and ease respiration. Little by little the lung loses its function as the one that clarifies and moves downward *qing su* 清肅 , and various symptoms of this loss appear.

> The lung masters the breaths of the grains of the five *zang*, and it does not receive their overlapping. Thus when there is emptiness, respiration is trying to find itself, and the breaths dwindle. When there is fullness, the chest is distended and breathing is labored.
>
> *Taisu*

The Kidneys store the Essences; the Essences are the dwelling place of the Will.
When the breaths of the Kidneys are empty, there is withdrawal.
When they are full, there is swelling, and the Five Zang know no peace. *(lines 115-117)*

> The Kidneys store the Will *zhi*.
>
> *Suwen*, Chapter 62

> The kidneys store the will. . . . When there is an overabundance of will, the belly is swollen and there is diarrhea of undigested food. When there is an insufficiency, there is a withdrawal *jue* 厥 .
>
> *Suwen*, Chapter 23

The kidneys store the essences and the will *jing zhi* 精志 .
Suwen, Chapter 78

The kidneys' thesaurization of the essences of the five *zang* is the base of power for the entire being, the rooting of the will. The very strength of memory and remembrance, of thoughts, of the brain — like the power of the bone structure and the posture of the body — depend on the richness of the essences of the kidneys.

The kidneys are thus linked to the origin, to the original *yin* and original *yang*.

Weakness in the kidneys is a decline of original *yang*; it is a diminishing of the deep solidity of life. One observes a growing colder, a generalized withdrawal, a lack of correct breaths and of the vital power, which now allows perverse breaths to intrude.

An overabundance of perverse breaths (perverse fullness) in the kidneys is an overflowing of water which causes bloating by accumulation. These bloatings may also come from a blockage of circulation in the lower belly, caused by the plethora of kidney breaths.

> The kidneys are the source of the breaths of life. This is why in emptiness the hands and feet grow cold through withdrawal *jue*. The kidneys are the gate-keeper of the stomach; when there is excess, the gateway of the defense no longer holds, and it gives way to swellings.
>
> *Zhang Zhicong*

The first case evokes the decline of original *yang*, which is first manifested at the extremities. Deserted by the breaths of life, the hands and feet turn cold and have no defense against the perverse breaths; this is withdrawal *jue*.

The second case evokes the circulation of the waters and their recovery, which is the charge and responsibility of the kidneys, especially in relation to the stomach (cf *Suwen*, Chapter 61). The swellings and bloatings are a sign of dysfunctioning kidneys due to blockage.

> The lung is the thesaurization of metal; it controls madness and withdrawal *kuang jue* 狂厥 . The kidneys are the thesaurization of water; they control the swelling due to water *shui zhang* 水脹. The Five *zang* are not at peace.

Metal begets water; thus when the son, water, is empty, the mother, metal, overlaps it; from this come madness and withdrawal in a counter-current.

Taisu

Taisu's commentary insists upon the mental aspect of withdrawal more than upon its physical aspect. The decline of vitality does not show simply through a chilling of the hands and feet, but also through a loss of consciousness and of the higher activities. Loss of reason or memory and all that ordinarily accompanies senility could be evoked here.

The sentence segment "the Five *Zang* know no peace" poses a problem. A certain number of classical commentators do not consider it the outcome of the account of the pathology of the excess of breaths of the kidneys. They prefer to attach it to the conclusion, which follows immediately after the statement about the kidneys. They would therefore make the following translation, combining the final phrase of line 117 with the sixth stanza, which is the conclusion. It should therefore be translated:

In the presence of this situation wherein the Five *Zang* know no peace, one must carefully discern the symptoms. . . .

This is the meaning: it is through the feelings, through internal disturbance of the wills, that the *zang* are no longer at peace and have symptoms of emptiness or fullness. One must diagnose these disturbances with as much exactness as possible in order to treat them and to re-balance the excess or deficiency of whatever *zang* one has singled out.

In contrast, if we place "the Five *Zang* know no peace" at the end of the pathology of excess kidney breaths, it must be understood that the kidneys, as with the spleen, pass on their imbalance to the whole of the *zang*.

With the kidneys it is no longer a question of loss of peace through lack or insufficiency, as it was for the spleen; it is a matter of a blockage, of an accumulation or congestion that blocks the kidneys from guaranteeing their role, and puts agitation, and possibly conflict, into the *zang* as a whole, which do not have the wherewithal of essences to be able to thesaurize peacefully.

It is notable that the spleen and kidneys provoke this disturbance of the loss of peace among the *zang*. Again we find the Anterior Heaven and Posterior Heaven coupling. We rediscover the two *zang* in charge of essences and in charge of supplying essences to the *zang*.

Conclusion: Uncontrolled Emotions Ruin Life

It will be necessary to discern with care the
symptoms of pathology of the Five **Zang,**
In order to be in a position to perceive the
emptiness or fullness of their breaths.
Be aware of this when you treat someone. (lines 118-120)

> The Dao of medical treatment is, first of all, to know the emptiness and fullness of the breaths of the five *zang* and to know which illnesses are produced by these emptinesses or fullnesses. Next, one prescribes treatment by needles or by medicines. Let us be careful when we treat.
>
> *Taisu*

The great teaching of this eighth chapter of the *Lingshu* is that a deep upset (through emptiness or through fullness) of each of the five *zang* may be provoked by a disturbance in the feelings, the wills, the Spirits. In the last analysis, all pathology is provoked, at its root, by a disturbance in the feelings, the wills, the Spirits.

The classical language plays fully on the radical opposition of terms. Rapid and sure, it flies toward its goal. It leaves to the theoreticians and practitioners of life the task of giving nuance, in concrete situations, to affirmations that are normally and regularly categorical. The text announces death tactlessly. In reality, if the lack of emotional control is brief, one risks the establishment of a tendency toward morbidity rather than a situation leading swiftly and ineluctably to death. We must, however, take very seriously the detailed warning addressed to us. If, through lightness of temperament, or momentary thoughtlessness, or careless passionate involvement, or debility due to age or to having arrived stealthily at the end of a pernicious illness, we allow ourselves to be led by our emotions on a long term basis, a day could well come where those emotions take us over, removing our power to control them. If the joy of life is lost and replaced by pessimism, we can find ourselves in the manacles and shackles of depression that we will have clasped upon ourselves.

This warning is the instruction given in the final part of Chapter 8 of *Lingshu*. It finds its natural place immediately after it has been established that "Knowing-how is the maintenance of life." In effect, the opposite of knowing-how and knowing-how-to-live is the incompetence of the ignorant who do not even know that the emotions must be controlled before they tyrannize us and cause our life to fall into ruins. What we have just read and commented upon is an "Art of Decline," which follows an "Art of Maintaining the Vital Principle" as its inverse image.

In the game of chess that is life, when the heart, which is king, is defended only by chessmen that are blocked or kept from moving, check becomes checkmate. The king is not taken, but the game is over. The lesson of this chapter, repeated throughout, is that we must not rush into all the possible gambits of the chess game, that we should not make a move without thinking, nor give in to anger, nor enjoy our momentary advantages too much. We must always guard our heart.

Appendices

The Thirteen Servants of Life and Death

In order to unify the thirteen ideas exposed separately and in detail in characters 84 to 186 (lines 17-30), we must consider the way the ideas are grouped, the stages of development they represent, and the way they form a hierarchy.

Just as Laozi (Chapter 50)[60] knows thirteen servants of life and death, Chapter 8 of the *Lingshu* cites thirteen instances[61] that contribute to the balance and conservation of a being's existence from the time of its emergence into life and its return into death. Man uses these thirteen companions for good or ill. In certain medical texts "the thirteen servants" can be interpreted to be the nine bodily orifices and the four limbs, representing different facets of internal and external human activity.

> These Thirteen, encountering man, strike a blow; and knowing-how is maintenance of life.
>
> *Ma Shi*

One can conserve life only with that which attacks it; the most beneficial currents return more powerfully against one who misuses them.

In approaching the totality of the thirteen aspects, one perceives two major divisions, each subdivided again into two sub-groups, as follows:

I. The first grouping of seven statements:

A. Virtue, Breaths, Life

(These retrace the great movement that is universal life.)

B. The Essences, The Spirits, The *Hun*, The *Po*

(These give to man's existence its spiritual dimension and invest it with powers beyond those involved in the simple evolution of human form between its appearance and disappearance.)

II. The last grouping of six statements:

A. The Heart, Intent, Will

(These are charged with the expression of the Spirits within man.)

B. Thought, Reflection, Knowing-how

(These enunciate the first specific expressions of man.)

---

[60] "One emerges, it is life; and returns, it is death
Thirteen are the companions of life.
Thirteen are the companions of death.
Moving one into the realms of death, the companions are also Thirteen."
[61] Aspects of life as well as stages of development.

GROUP I.A: *Virtue, Breaths, Life*

The primordial couple (Heaven/Earth) is an image of all couples and all couplings. In between them there is life and living beings.

Nothing specifically "human" appears here, except that Virtue is reflected in the human heart, and that the breaths are reflected in all the perpetually changing elements of the human's vitality and vivacity. This triplicity is associated both with cosmic, universal life, and with the life of every living being. It connects that which forms an individual "me" to the more general life of the Universe.

GROUP I.B: *The Essences, the Spirits, the* **Hun***, the* **Po** *(The Rooting in the Spirits)*

These four statements give form to human evolution, to the ungraspable aspects of life, and to the mystery of life within man. There are two couples: Essences/Spirits *jing/shen* 精神 , and the *Hun/po* 魂魄. The second couple is closely subordinated to the first, and each of its terms defined in connection with the terms of the first couple. The *Hun* exist only through the Spirits and in their rapport with the Spirits, and the *Po* exist only with the Essences.

In Group I.A. we have Heaven and Earth manifesting through Virtue and Breaths, and then Life. In Group I.B., first we have the Essences and the Spirits taking up life at the level of a living being who is beginning to be expressed and take form. In the couple, Essences/Spirits, the *yin* Essences precede the *yang* Spirits. Subordinate to these come the couple, the *Hun* and Po. Here the order of *yin* and *yang* is reversed in order to show that which is connected to the *yang* principle (the *Hun*), before that which is tied to the *yin* (the Po). *Jing shen* (Essences/Spirits) and *hun po*, are the usual order in which these terms are given, and this recalls at every instant the ceaseless interconnections of Life. Man does not choose his essences or his Spirits; it is they who make him what he is. The *hun* and *po* are more dependent upon him, in the sense that their strength or weakness (and thus the length of their life) depends in part on the life he leads. But *hun* and *po* are nevertheless beyond ephemeral existence.

The essences, like the Spirits, dwell outside of time and substance. However, they are the condition of all material expression, spatial and temporal. The *hun* and *po* are temporalized at the level of life on earth and beyond; they are restricted within time. The *hun* and *po* are also more "materialized" than the Essences/Spirits: one can call forth the *hun*, or evoke and feel their presence in, for example, a sacrifice to the ancestors; the *po* are feared, as they can take possession of a living being or simply become manifest in the form of an apparition or a ghost. In ancient times *hun* and *po* were certainly endowed with the power to intervene in our affairs, including the preservation of life or the loss of life.

Style

By their number, the three[62] statements making up the first sub-group (I.A) can represent the animation that is as yet undifferentiated by the breaths, which are still the Breath, that is, not yet the precise breaths of a being or a species. This Breath is at the origin and root of life of the one hundred species of each of the Ten Thousand Beings.

By their number, the four statements making up the second sub-group (I.B) can show the constituted presence of the highest level of animation. This level is nearest "the ancestors" of life who, alone, endure (eternally).

Looking at the presentation of the lines of Chinese characters (characters 84-186, following lines 17-30 of the English text), we see that a subtle play on the number of characters composing each statement helps us feel the progression of the process of incarnation.

The first two statements (lines 14 and 15 in the Chinese characters) have an equal number of characters (seven each), and the third statement (line 16) has one more (making eight). This emphasizes the sudden appearance of life.

If we put aside the particle *gu* 故 (thus), which nonetheless has meaning in the whole passage, each of the four succeeding statements increases by one character the length of the preceding one: the fourth statement giving a definition of essences contains six characters, not including *gu*; the fifth statement contains seven; the sixth statement contains eight; the seventh statement contains nine. The lengthening of the presentation corresponds to the descent into incarnation.

---

[62] Three is the proper number for breaths, and four is the proper number for the form given by Earth to things and beings.

GROUP II.A. *The Heart, Intent, Will*
(The Heart Proposes and Disposes)

The heart is the great pivot of the text. It is the eighth of the thirteen aspects, calling to mind the whirlwind of the eight winds that occupy all available space and time to deliver the presence of life everywhere.

The heart marks man's arrival at self-possession and at the mastery of his destiny, his future. Intent, will, thought, and reflection are all written with the radical for the heart ⺁心 : they are the effects created by the power of the Spirits moving through the heart.

With the heart, it is a question of man's life and that alone. At death nothing remains of the heart, and nothing remains of its servants and messengers.

From this moment on we see that the treasures of the five *zang* – Spirits (heart), Essences (kidneys), *Hun* (liver), *Po* (lung), Intent (spleen), and Will (kidneys) – can be referred to on the same scheme only if one distinguishes the levels carefully.

It is essential to put in its appropriate place the appearance of the Heart, which is the same as a taking of responsibility. The following "authorities" (differentiated functions) may rather easily be variously attached to one or another *zang*. Intent (and also Thought) may be associated with the spleen, the Will with the kidneys, Reflection with the liver, and Knowing-how with the spleen or kidneys. However, we are not concerned with these relationships, but with the flourishing they give to the heart.

> Of all these many notions, each is mastered (controlled) by a particular *zang*; however, all are born in the heart, for all the *zang* are only auxiliaries and agents *xiang shi* 相使, and the heart is the supreme master, the absolute chief *zhu zai* 主宰
>
> *Zhang Jiebin*

> All of that is the effects coming from the movement of distribution of the influx of the heart's Spirits; that is why knowing-how is following the nature of Heaven/Earth, possessing it and thus maintaining the Way of life.
>
> *Zhang Zhicong*

Intent and Will are nearest to the heart, the most closely attached, the heart's intimates. Intent and Will structure the person's own particular animation. They must be in harmony to assure good order and fair control or else the heart loses its way; Intent and Will get disconnected and disorganized, and there is disorder and trouble. We cannot say that Will and Intent are good or bad: either they exercise a regulatory control, or they show themselves incapable of doing so.

"The five authorities," usually presented as that which is stored by the five *zang*, have all been named. They are Spirits, *Hun*, *Po*, Intent, and Will (or essences, both relating to the kidneys). We postulate that it is impossible to place them in the creative cycle (*sheng*) or the control cycle (*ke*) of the Five Elements. We also postulate that they are in a continuous chain where the heart holds a special place between the Spirits that go beyond earthly destiny (*shen, hun, po*) and the means by which the individual controls and directs that destiny (intent and will). We postulate, therefore, a double presence, equally of the heart (in the form of Spirits and in the form of the heart) and of the kidneys (in the form of essences and in the form of will). The explanation for this is as follows: in a Being the kidneys are double; they are the symbolic receptacles of the origin of life (this will be specified in later works of the Chinese Tradition by the name *ming men* 命門 , Water and Fire, the authentic and original *yin* and *yang*), and they are linked to the essences in a privileged way. The kidneys, one of the five *zang*, connected to the water element, are also the seat of the will.

Similarly, the heart is double: as the ungraspable void, placed within non-form and non-action *wu wei* 無為 ,[63] it is the dwelling place of the Spirits; or it is the heart taking charge of ruling over life, and giving rise to intent, will, and thought.

From a metric point of view, let us count the number of characters in each statement: the statement presenting the heart contains eight characters; the statements relative to purpose and will each have seven. We find equality and symmetry in the presentation of intent and will: three ideograms are the same, and are found in the same place in each of the two lines – *suo* 所 and *wei zhi* 謂之.

---

[63] Non-interference.

GROUP II.B: *Thought, Reflection, Knowing-how (The Conduct of Life)*

Thought, reflection and knowing-how are modes of conduct and movements that may be perverted. When perverted, thought becomes involuted and folds back upon itself, reiterating indefinitely, repeating itself tirelessly. Reflection becomes uncertainty, anxiety, fear, and doubt. There is no more knowing-how — only artifice and stratagems.

These movements are presented in three statements of eight characters each. There are strict parallels in all three statements: four common characters in identical places — *yin* 因 , *er* 而 , *wei zhi* 謂之.

From intent expressed through will, we can indefinitely draw the authorities, the feelings and emotions of life. Here, thought and consciousness lead to knowing; farther along in this discussion the passions, which affect the will, lead us to analyses of the pathology of emotions.

Logic of the Text [64]

The complete logical analysis of the text requires study of the particles. To avoid overburdening our own commentaries we shall not do that here, despite our interest in such work. However, for those who want to be aware of the articulations of thought, we propose a brief interpretation of several "empty" characters, that is, particles of liaison and subordination, limiting our interpretation to the meanings they assume in this text.

> **Zhe** 者 : an enclitic, uniting with the preceding character to form one unit, taken as a whole. Or it simply underlines the object of discourse or marks a pause.
>
> **Ye** 也 : final particle, most often underlining an affirmation.
>
> **Zhi** 之 : a determining article, or a genitive, or a possessive; it can also underline a word.
>
> **Wei** 謂 : to say, to signify, to mean, to name, to be.
>
> **Wei zhi** 謂之: "given what has just been stated, one can say . . ."

---

[64] This section will be of interest to those readers who are studying Chinese characters.

> *Yin* 因 : "relying on what has just been stated, one can infer from it that ..." From here comes the meaning of: because of, as a result of.
> *Gu* 故 : therefore, that is why, consequently.
> *Suo yi* 所以: that by means of which, that by which.

GROUP I.A: there is no introductory particle, but a final one, the particle *ye*: emphatic support, a pause.

GROUP I.B: introduced by *gu*, procession of particular consequences: it is the organization of the human.

GROUP II.A: introduced by *suo yi*: unfolds the more limited life that flows out of the first conditions and functions.

GROUP II.B: each of the three propositions is introduced by a *yin*: these are the induced effects.

Let us go over each of the groups in deeper detail:

GROUP I.A.

In lines one and two, *zhe* 者 after *wo* 我 (I, me) underlines and reinforces by reuniting the preceding ensemble of characters into a whole. In these ensembles, *zhi* 之 underlines Heaven (line one) or Earth (line two).

In line three, *zhe* 者 after *sheng* 生 , life, puts the accent on the living "me."

This living being is the vessel, the visibility of the great cosmic powers. These powers are presented "in me," active and reflected in an ego, which allows us to grasp them at the human level where we are, the only level that we can immediately apprehend. Life *sheng* is the supreme cosmic result in the absolute beginning of a "me" *wo*.

The first two *zhe* introduce a clarification and place Virtue in relationship with Heaven ("in me"), and the Breaths in relationship with Earth ("in me"); whereas the third *zhe* is final. The *zhe* followed by a *ye*, *zhe ye* 者也 , is the musical pause: life is the supreme and definitive happening. That which constitutes and reconstitutes life is observed through life and through a living being. Let us not try to establish whether the chicken came before the egg. Let us look at life, and let us live.

GROUP I.B.

This group is introduced by *gu* 故 . The group signifies arrival at the level of the existence of particular beings. Let us see which chicken the egg comes from, and what this egg is.

Having stepped into the domain of particulars, we are content to describe the generation of the authorities of life, one after the other. Thus the use of *wei* 謂 : the manifested may be designated in such and such a way. *Wei* completed by *zhi* 之 perfects and firmly fixes the significance. By contrast, in none of the propositions of Group A is there a designation or a name, *wei*.

Lines 17 and 18 are the pure movement of life: a coming (an appearance) then a grasping, an embrace. These are movements indicating the essences and the Spirits.

In lines 19 and 20, reality is more perceptible; *zhe* 者 , *that which* is going to execute such a movement or such an action, is spoken of here. Thus the *hun* and the *po* appear.

GROUP II.A.

The heart appears in the same way as the *hun* and the *po*: it is the one that takes responsibility.

But throughout the repetition of the same formula, *zhe wei zhi* 者謂之 , there is a gulf between the presentation of the *hun* and the *po*, and that of the heart. In the presentation of the heart, the remarkable and unique fact is that nothing from the preceding text is repeated. The heart takes the eighth position (the number of the chapter, the number of winds . . .). Everything is distributed from the heart, especially the calm and still winds or the impetuous and violent winds of the feelings and passions.

In introducing Group II.A., the expression *suo yi* 所以 marks a rupture while at the same time creating a bond. Out of the preceding, the heart exists. Because of what precedes, life is in a responsible and living "I." Essences, Spirits, *hun*, *po* — that which I am — support my life, allow me to survive, bathe me in this life that surrounds me on every side, and erase the boundaries of time and space. Thus the life that is me specifies its commandment, grants the power to accomplish the "mandate" *ming* 命 of nature, and lays out the journey. That life is the heart.

The heart is formed as "the one who" takes on the task. The authorities that come after the statement of the heart's position consist simply of the expression *wei zhi* 謂之 . They note the movements of the heart.

The heart is Emperor, the sacred vessel of the Empire. Intent and will *yi zhi* 意志、 are its direct ministers (like those who stand to the left and the right of the Emperor).

GROUP II.B.

Starting from the will, a cascade of logical effects *yin* 因 shows thought, reflection, and knowing-how flowing from one to the other, each relying on the preceding one and on the entire preceding ensemble.

Thought and reflection are the government cabinet for deliberations and decisions. Knowing-how is the radiance of the Sovereign. Thus knowing is the effect of reflection and, through all that precedes it, it is the effect of the heart. Thus all the ideograms following the heart contain its radical 心 , except for the last one, knowing-how: it proceeds from the heart, but what matters is that it objectively reaches all beings *wu* 物 , including all immediate components of its own being, its own "me." In knowing-how *zhi* 智, what is in the heart is now poured forth.

It is said that the Empire is "under Heaven," between Heaven and Earth. It is alive, filled with the Spirits of Heaven and of Earth *gui shen* 鬼神, which must be respected and maintained in their place (cf. Laozi, ch. 60). The Empire is full of all the natural resources, correctly and cleverly handled and divided up. The ancestors are present above the people. Such is the life of the Empire. That life surpasses the empire of the moment and whatever dynasty happens to be ruling. In the matter of the Empire, Heaven/Earth itself fulfills the Mandate. The majesty of the Chinese throne stems from its being occupied by the Son of Heaven[65] (for instance Huangdi, the Yellow Emperor), for Heaven has given its Son the power to govern humankind.

---

[65] Traditionally a name for all the Emperors of China.

Concordance Wade, Pinyin

Wade	Pinyin		Wade	Pinyin
a	a		chui	zhui
ai	ai		ch'ui	chui
an	an		chun	zhun
ang	ang		ch'un	chun
ao	ao		chung	zhong
cha	zha		ch'ung	chong
ch'a	cha		chü	ju
chai	zhai		ch'ü	qu
ch'ai	chai		chüan	juan
chan	zhan		ch'üan	quan
ch'an	chan		chüeh	jue
chang	zhang		ch'üeh	que
ch'ang	chang		chün	jun
chao	zhao		ch'ün	qun
ch'ao	chao		e	e
che	zhe		ei	ei
ch'e	che		en	en
chen	zhen		erh	erh
ch'en	chen		fa	fa
cheng	zheng		fan	fan
ch'eng	cheng		fang	fang
chi	ji		fei	fei
ch'i	qi		fen	fen
chia	jia		feng	feng
ch'ia	qia		fo	fo
chiang	jiang		fou	fou
ch'iang	qiang		fu	fu
chiao	jiao		ha	ha
ch'iao	qiao		hai	hai
chieh	jie		han	han
ch'ieh	qie		hang	hang
chien	jian		hao	hao
ch'ien	qian		he	he
chih	zhi		hei	hei
ch'ih	chi		hen	hen
chin	jin		heng	heng
ch'in	qin		ho	he
ching	jing		hou	hou
ch'ing	qing		hsi	xi
chiu	jiu		hsia	xia
ch'iu	qiu		hsiang	xiang
chiung	jiong		hsiao	xiao
ch'iung	qiong		hsieh	xie
cho	zhuo		hsien	xian
ch'o	chuo		hsin	xin
chou	zhou		hsing	xing
ch'ou	chou		hsiu	xiu
chu	zhu		hsiung	xiong
ch'u	chu		hsü	xu
chua	zhua		hsüan	xuan
chuai	zhuai		hsüeh	xue
ch'uai	chuai		hsün	xun
chuan	zhuan		hu	hu
ch'uan	chuan		hua	hua
chuang	zhuang		huai	huai
ch'uang	chuang		huan	huan

Wade	Pinyin	Wade	Pinyin
huang	huang	la	la
hui	hui	lai	lai
hun	hun	lan	lan
hung	hong	lang	lang
huo	huo	lao	lao
i	yi	le	le
jan	ran	lei	lei
jang	rang	leng	leng
jao	rao	li	li
je	re	lia	lia
jen	ren	liang	liang
jeng	reng	liao	liao
jih	ri	lieh	lie
jo	ruo	lien	lian
jou	rou	lin	lin
ju	ru	ling	ling
juan	ruan	liu	liu
jui	rui	lo	luo
jun	run	lou	lou
jung	rong	lu	lu
ka	ga	luan	luan
k'a	ka	lun	lun
kai	gai	lung	long
k'ai	kai	lü	lü
kan	gan	lüan	lüan
k'an	kan	lüeh	lüe
kang	gang	ma	ma
k'ang	kang	mai	mai
kao	gao	man	man
k'ao	kao	mang	mang
ke (ko)	ge	mao	mao
k'e (k'o)	ke	mei	mei
ken	gen	men	men
k'en	ken	meng	meng
keng	geng	mi	mi
k'eng	keng	miao	miao
kou	gou	mieh	mie
k'ou	kou	mien	mian
ku	gu	min	min
k'u	ku	ming	ming
kua	gua	miu	miu
k'ua	kua	mo	mo
kuai	guai	mou	mou
k'uai	kuai	mu	mu
kuan	guan	na	na
k'uan	kuan	nai	nai
kuang	guang	nan	nan
k'uang	kuang	nang	nang
kuei	gui	nao	nao
k'uai	kui	ne	ne
kun	gun	nei	nei
k'un	kun	nen	nen
kung	gong	neng	neng
k'ung	kong	ni	ni
kuo	guo	niang	niang
k'uo	kuo	niao	niao

Wade	Pinyin	Wade	Pinyin
nieh	nie	shai	shai
nien	nian	shan	shan
nin	nin	shang	shang
ning	ning	shao	shao
niu	niu	she	she
no	nuo	shei	shei
nou	nou	shen	shen
nu	nu	sheng	sheng
nuan	nuan	shih	shi
nung	nong	shou	shou
nü	nü	shu	shu
nüeh	nüe	shua	shua
ou	ou	shuai	shuai
pa	ba	shuan	shuan
p'a	pa	shuang	shuang
pai	bai	shui	shui
p'ai	pai	shun	shun
pan	ban	shuo	shuo
p'an	pan	so	suo
pang	bang	sou	sou
p'ang	pang	su	su
pao	bao	suan	suan
p'ao	pao	sui	sui
pei	bei	sun	sun
p'ei	pei	sung	song
pen	ben	szu	si
p'en	pen	ta	da
peng	beng	t'a	ta
p'eng	peng	tai	dai
pi	bi	t'ai	tai
p'i	pi	tan	dan
piao	biao	t'an	tan
p'iao	piao	tang	dang
pieh	bie	t'ang	tang
p'ieh	pie	tao	dao
pien	bian	t'ao	tao
p'ien	pian	te	de
pin	bin	t'e	te
p'in	pin	teng	deng
ping	bing	t'eng	teng
p'ing	ping	ti	di
po	bo	t'i	ti
p'o	po	tiao	diao
p'ou	pou	t'iao	tiao
pu	bu	tieh	die
p'u	pu	t'ieh	tie
sa	sa	tien	dian
sai	sai	t'ien	tian
san	san	ting	ding
sang	sang	t'ing	ting
sao	sao	tiu	diu
se	se	to	duo
sen	sen	t'o	tuo
seng	seng	tou	dou
sha	sha	t'ou	tou

Wade	Pinyin	Wade	Pinyin
tsa	za	t'uan	tuan
ts'a	ca	tui	dui
tsai	zai	t'ui	tui
ts'ai	cai	tun	dun
tsan	zan	t'un	tun
ts'an	can	tung	dong
tsang	zang	t'ung	tong
ts'ang	cang	tzu	zi
tsao	zao	tz'u	ci
ts'ao	cao	wa	wa
tse	ze	wai	wai
ts'e	ce	wan	wan
tsei	zei	wang	wang
tsen	zen	wei	wei
ts'en	cen	wen	wen
tseng	zeng	weng	weng
ts'eng	ceng	wo	wo
tso	zuo	wu	wu
ts'o	cuo	ya	ya
tsou	zou	yai	yai
ts'ou	cou	yang	yang
tsu	zu	yao	yao
ts'u	cu	yeh	ye
tsuan	zuan	yen	yan
ts'uan	cuan	yin	yin
tsui	zui	ying	ying
ts'ui	cui	yo	yo
tsun	zun	yu	you
ts'un	cun	yung	yong
tsung	zong	yü	yu
ts'ung	cong	yüan	yuan
tu	du	yüeh	yue
t'u	tu	yün	yun
tuan	duan		

Glossary

Note: *In each heading, the* pinyin *Romanization of the Chinese character will be given first, followed by the Wade-Giles transliteration placed in parentheses. Where there are no parentheses following the* pinyin, *it is because the two are the same.*

Anger   Nu

In one's heart 心 one has the frustrated feeling of an enslaved woman 女 over whom someone has the upper hand 又 . This is anger *nu*.

Anger is thus something that bursts out as well as something that remains buried and turned within. When the accumulated pressure explodes, blood and breaths are taken massively toward the upper regions. When it is held inside, the internal agitation and dissatisfaction generate blockages that have no resolution. Blocked situations that have no resolution eat away at us.

Anger corresponds to the liver. When it expresses the normality of the Wood element, it is the very impetuosity of life, especially in the power of things at their beginning. It is the strength of wind that blows, or the young plant breaking through the still-frozen ground, or the fierceness of birth that expels a being into the light of day and then causes it to grow and unfurl. Wind is the "anger" of Heaven.

Pathological anger is perverse movement of the Wood. This is the force that unleashes impulses and pushes them to their extreme; it is the upward leap, the impetuosity that carries everything along before it. When it breaks its moorings, leaves its roots, and goes out of control, it is rage, unleashed fury, and irrational anger.

Breaths   Qi(Ch'i)

Breaths are vapor, exhalation, fluid, influx, and energies, vital life force.

The grain of rice 米 that bursts with cooking or digestion releases a vapor that rises up and accumulates 气 .

Breaths themselves are formless, but they produce, animate, and maintain all form. They draw strength and renewal from the work that is carried out on all transformable matter.

Everything is made by the breaths. It is not the quantity of breaths that makes health; it is the harmonious distribution of all the components that must go, by themselves, to the places where they are expected.

The circulations and exchanges, the changes from liquid into vapor and from vapor into liquid, the rhythms of movements, and the openings and closings of countless gates and orifices in the body all occur thanks to the breaths.

Clarity Qing
(Ch'ing)

Pure and regenerative 青 water 水. It is what rises and diffuses, thanks to its lightness and subtlety.

Elation & Joy Xi Le
(Hsi Le)

喜 樂

Xi. A hand strikes the skin of a drum 壴 , and the mouth 口 allows joyful songs to burst forth. This is the pleasure of village festivals, the excitement of singing and dancing to the frenetic sound of the little drum. This is elation.

Le. The large drum 白 , framed by resonances (bells or lithophones) 幺 , is mounted on a wooden stand 木 . This is joy, the official music which is orderly and, at court, marks rhythmically the ceremonies and life of the Empire. The rhythmic beat is powerful but never unrestrained.

In elation there is excitation, something lively and light, in the image of a hand beating drums rapidly and rhythmically. The vital dynamism bursts and is manifested with youthful exuberance in the thrust of hot, red blood.

Joy is calmer than elation. In joy there is slowness, depth, tranquillity, harmony, and concerted and orchestrated vibration. In Chinese the same character is used for joy and for music.

When elation and joy are allied, *joie de vivre* is displayed. It is born from the movements of breaths whose ordered circulation gives an impulse that is unified in the heart and by the heart.

Elation and joy correspond to the heart. In their negative aspect, they are the perversion of the Fire movement. Fire radiates and warms, so that the effects of blossoming and the expansion of the free and easy circulation and communications can be felt in all parts of one's being. If the Fire gets carried away, everything bursts forth from everywhere and is propelled toward the periphery, toward empty air, toward the far distance. If joy gets carried away, well-being imperceptibly becomes excitation. No longer under control, *yang* displays its effects which enchant, because it is the most natural movement of life. But it exhausts and wastes itself, leaving the being collapsed and dazed, not knowing from where this disenchantment comes.

Emotions

情

Qing (Ch'ing)

The heart 心 and the greenery of ascending life 青 . This signifies that the emotions, which are the interior dispositions of a being, are good when they occur naturally and harmful when they become passions.

Essences

精

Jing
(Ch'ing)

The choicest grain which is refined, elite, and subtle. It is the quintessence, or the most perfect embodiment of something.

To the bursting and decomposing grain of rice or millet 米, present in the writing of the character 氣 (*qi*, breaths), we add greenery rather than the rising of steam that is in the character for *qi*.

Greenery is *qing* 青, the color of a growing plant 生 pushed upward by rich sap, its fluid of life 丹. This can be green, or any color showing a living being's vitality distributed to the most exterior regions.

The pure and clear essences are the template for each life (essences of Anterior Heaven received from the mother and the father), and they are the basis for that life's maintenance and continuation (essences of Posterior Heaven received from food and air). The essences pass from one being to another (in food, for example), through decomposition (as in digestion) and through assimilation. By mutual resonance the essences reach the *zang* which they regenerate and where they are "worked." They are the materials full of vitality that weave all living things.

There are also:

Essences/
Breaths

精 氣

Jing Qi
(Ching Ch'i)

Essences and breaths constitute the crucible wherein life is created and maintained. The essences give themselves to the transformations in order to start up the breaths. The breaths resulting from the transformations of the essences are the breaths of the deep, authentic life of a being. Transformations *hua* 化 are the effects of the breaths working on the essences.

Essences/ Spirits
精神

Jing Shen (Ching Shen)

Jing Shen is the vital Spirit, the animating Spirits of the essence. It is human vitality at its most subtle level of expression. It is the active totality of life active for life's clear and conscious governance. The essences fasten the Spirits in place and give them a way to be expressed. The Spirits free the subtlety of the essences for the higher operations of life.

Fear & Fright
恐懼

Kong Ju (K'ung Chu)

Kong. The beating heart 心 subjected to repeated blows, as when one builds a structure 工 by re. eated strokes, by small blows of a hammer 丸 . This is fear, to be frightened, to dread.

Ju. The internal feeling in the heart 心 is like the picture of small birds 隹 opening their fearful eyes 䀠 to maintain the vigilance necessary for their safety. There is fear, anxiety, dread.

Fear is the rupture of beneficial communication between above and below, between the heart and the kidneys. The Spirits of the heart, no longer enjoying support from the kidney essences, go astray, and their conduct becomes unconscious. The breaths, blocked or insufficient, provoke palpitations. Deprived of dynamism, the essences no longer rise, no longer hold together, and one becomes empty from below.

When the blows have disorganized the connections between Water and Fire, either brusquely or little by little, essences and breaths withdraw, each to their own territory in the trunk of the body: essences below, and breaths above, in the trunk of the body. Thus there may be agitated fear and headlong flight, or feverishness and permanent panic.

When the Breaths or the Fire are weak, the movement of Water, which now draws downward and freezes, is no longer balanced and gradually takes over all the levels of one's being. Then there is insecurity and hesitation, and one is nailed to the spot, immobile, paralyzed.

Fear, which corresponds to the kidneys, is a perversion of the movement of Water. Water is a controlled attraction downward that solidly maintains the foundations of life. Fear is an unrestrained sinking, an uncontrolled descent.

Fear thus invades the liver and the Wood, which can now no longer find the wherewithal for launching themselves from what has become a deficient base (kidneys, Water). Fear, then, opposes the impetuous ardor of the liver and the male courage of the Gall Bladder.

Finally, the heart fire will be unable to radiate as a consequence of successive weakenings due to this hunching downward. One crouches, hiding, no longer revealing oneself to the light, and the light no longer appears.

Fu

腑

Organs/ Bowels

Depot, warehouse, residence, bowels.

The six *Fu* are the temporary depositories where alimentation is made assimilable through transformations, and where the essences (that which can be assimilated) are directed toward the interior of the body and the wastes evacuated to the exterior. The Six *Fu* sift and sort, assigning to each part its useful destination. The fact that there are Six denotes the circulations and exchanges with which they are charged for the vital maintenance. These are the exchanges between the interior and the exterior, the circulation from the upper to the lower parts of the trunk, and assimilation and elimination.

Heart   Xin (Hsin)

The written form of the character for the heart 心 is often turned around to give this form 忄. The following sequence of strokes show how this change has come about: 心 忄 忄 忄 忄

Heart, spirit, intimacy, intelligence, thought, mentality, moral conscience, feeling, emotion, humor, intention, and attention.

The heart 心 represents man's heart: the open pericardium above; the organ in the middle; and below, a brief indication of the aorta

Open at the top, the heart is permanently penetrated by the influx descending from above; it communicates with Heaven through the Spirits.

At the center, there is nothing but emptiness, the only possible shelter for the Spirits. Sovereign of the being and pivot of life, the heart is the guarantor of the unity of a person's existence.

Communications are established below, toward the other organic authorities. The heart thus radiates its influence and transmits its orders. The blood is the bearer, *par excellence*, of the heart's orders.

As Absolute Sovereign, the heart is also one of the Five *Zang*, expressing the movement appropriate to the Fire, the flame that rises. The Fire dispenses a soft warmth that stimulates the infinite circulation of life, rising up from the depths, spreading out, and filling all of space. As Sovereign, the heart is master of the five *Zang* and the six *Fu*, of all the emotions, and of all the upper orifices. As a *zang* expressing one of the five aspects of the vital movement, it particularizes the Fire, the brightness of summer's maturation and ripening, and the *yang* expansion of life in the south. The heart conserves permanently this double aspect.

The circulation of the blood under the heart's authority carries regularly, everywhere, the double maintenance of life, which is both nutritive and spiritual. It reconstitutes vitality while also permitting sensitivity and the going and coming of information between the inside and the outside. The quality of blood and its governance by proportioned breaths are judged by the pulsations of the network of animation, which are the pulses, and by the color of the face (complexion).

The tongue, orifice of the heart, distinguishes the flavors but also expresses judgments (that which has come to consciousness in the heart, where things in the memory intersect with external stimulation and information).

The ear, which is another orifice of the heart, indicates this aptitude for receiving and picking up information.

> The heart is given the charge of being Lord and master. The luminous radiance of the Spirits proceeds from there. . . .
>
> *Suwen*, Chapter 8

> The heart is the trunk where life is rooted, and the place where the Spirits assure the changes. Its flowering aspect is the face; the power of its fullness is in the blood circulating through the network of animation. It is the great *yang* within *yang*, in free communication with the breaths of summer.
>
> *Suwen*, Chapter 9

> The southern quadrant generates heat. Heat generates fire. Fire generates bitter. Bitter generates the heart. The heart generates blood. Blood generates the spleen. The heart has mastery over the tongue. . . . In the bodily structures it is the network of animation. . . . Among the colors it is red. Among the musical notes it is the note *zhi*. Among the sounds it is laughter. Among the reactive movements to change it is oppression.
>
> *Suwen*, Chapter 5

> It opens its orifice at the eye. . . . Its domestic animal is the sheep. Its grain is glutinous millet. . . . Its odor is scorched.
>
> *Suwen*, Chapter 4

Hun

The *Hun* are spiritual souls, rational Spirits, the soul breath.

They are the Earthly Spirits 鬼 , animated by the same movement as the clouds 云 .

The Earthly Spirits *gui* 鬼 are contraposed to the Heavenly Spirits *shen* 神 . Earthly Spirits are represented by a head 白 above something that is more a vaporous form than a body 儿 , with an appendage ム symbolizing the whirlwind that accompanies the movement of Earthly Spirits (which can also be ghosts) but which also evokes a hook, representing the avidity of unassuaged demons in snatching living quarry.

Clouds 云 result from humidity pulled from Earth by the heat and by the attraction of Heaven. Clouds move freely at the will of the breaths in the celestial vault, spreading their beneficial shadows over the Earth.

As the clouds move, so move the *Hun*, as well as the shades of the ancestors.

Their dwelling place in the body is the liver (see Liver).

(See also *Po*)

Intent   Yi

意   (I)

Meaning, significance, intention, idea, opinion, personal feeling.

The intention of the heart 心 that the thinking, speaking, and acting person puts into what he emits 音 in sounds, thoughts, or acts.

The musical note *yin* 音 is a celestial vibration, a quality that Heaven confers upon a breath produced by a being.

By adding a specific graphic part on to the left of the character *yi*, we shift and show the multiple facets of the meaning of *yi*, for a better understanding.

憶 *Yi* : to apply oneself; intent 意 arising in the heart 心 ; to remember, to recall to one's spirit, to apply one's heart and one's thought to something. It is the application of the heart that takes into account what comes and presents itself.

億 *Yi* : a person's 人 = (亻) intent 意 ; a calm and peaceful atmosphere; the possibility of appreciating in a just way; to foresee exactly and to provide to each according to his need, indefinitely.

臆 *Yi* : the location of intent 意 in a fleshly body 肉 = 月 is the chest, the seat of the intelligence, of awareness, of feelings, and of personal opinions and viewpoints.

藝 *Yi* : intent 意 in the vegetable world 屮屮 = (艹) is the heart of the lotus seed, the intimate place from which the multiplicity of petals proceeds, the command center from which the corolla opens.

(See also Will)

Kidneys   Shen

Within the realm of the flesh 肉 , the kidneys are analagous to the firmness of a master whose hand 又 knows how to hold people 臣 wisely and solidly.

The kidneys are the foundation of life, repositories of Water and Fire, and of *yin* and *yang* whose embrace bring about the beginning of a being.

The kidneys present both a *yin* and a *yang* aspect: they draw down into the depths, but they do so in order to re-emerge. They are the guarantee of the fertile union of *yin* and *yang* in a being, like the union between the marrow and the bone. The marrow, held inside the bones, assures the power and the smooth suppleness of the bone, and the bone itself prevents the dissipation of the essential richness of the marrow. It is like the joining of two beings at the time of sexual union. The kidneys are sometimes taken for their original value, sometimes for the aspect of the vital movement that they represent — that of the Water.

This vital movement of the water is twofold: on the one hand it draws powerfully into the depths, for fertilization; on the other, it gently offers itself to all the metamorphoses: evaporation taking water to the heights; evacuation ejecting it below. Water lends itself to all of life's uses, on condition that the breaths, and also the Fire, be there to transform and move it perpetually.

The kidneys guard and work the essences, so that they may remain faithful to themselves, at their origin, and so that they may perpetuate the vitality throughout all the *zang*. The kidneys give the fundamental strength to the being via the essences; by their transformations they produce marrow, which sustains the vertical posture and gives strength to the brain as well as to the bones. The kidneys produce sperm, the origin of a new life. They give solidity to the teeth and softness to the hair on the head. Their orifices are either for receiving above (the ear), or for evacuation below (the two lower orifices).

Below, they sustain life by guarding what is essential and original, thus permitting the deployment of the most visible effects of animation.

The kidneys are given the charge of arousing the power.
Cleverness and ingenuity come from them.

Suwen, Chapter 8

The kidneys are the trunk (foundation) of whatever both masters hibernation and seals the storage of treasure (thesaurization). They are the residence of the essences. Their flowering aspect is the head hair, and the power of their fullness is in the bones. They are young *yin* within *yin*, in free communication with the breaths of winter.

Suwen, Chapter 9

The northern quadrant generates cold. Cold generates water. Water generates the salty taste. The salty taste generates the kidneys. The kidneys generate bones and marrow. Marrow generates the liver. The kidneys have mastery over the ear. . . . Among the colors they are soot-black. Among the musical notes they are the note *yu*. Among the sounds they are heavy sighing. Among the reactive movements to change they are shivering.

Suwen, Chapter 5

They open their orifice at the two *yin* (lower orifices). . . .
Their domestic animal is the pig; their cereal is the pea. . . .
Their odor is fermented.

Suwen, Chapter 4

The kidneys command water and receive the essences of
the five *zang* and the six *fu* in order to thesaurize them.

Suwen, Chapter 1

Knowing-How

智

Zhi
(Chih)

Intelligence, wisdom, prudence, talent, capacity.

The character is knowledge (awareness) 知 above the sun 日 , or
— according to other sources — knowledge above the word coming forth
from a mouth 曰 . In either case, the lower part expresses the
manifestation of power.

The upper part, knowledge, represents an arrow 矢 and a mouth 口 .
The arrow's precision gives the capability to speak about a subject, by
going straight to the goal. Knowledge/awareness is exact perception.
One knows something because one has gained precise awareness of it
(through the sense organs), one conceives what it is (in the heart), and
one can express it (via the tongue and the mouth) and manifest it (by
one's light).

When one has considered everything profoundly and intelligently,
and when each thing and each being has been appreciated at its true
value and is in its place in thought and in the plan, the heart is at ease.
It can express itself and radiate its light.

When one really knows, one knows what to do and how to do it. One
makes a just decision and acts efficaciously, and life is powerful.

> The spirit of discernment is the rule of prudence (knowing-
> how).
>
> Mencius

Life, Living Beings

Sheng

生

To live, to bring to life, to be born, to grow, to engender, and to produce. Life, living beings, a native state, vitality, and length of life.

A sprout 屮 , full of sap, grows and pushes up 出 vigorously 生 . Every living thing, whether plant or man, has the virtue and the uprightness necessary to lift itself toward Heaven while keeping its roots, drawing up the multiple resources from the Earth and spreading its branches right and left without losing vigor, until its demise.

This is the upward thrust of life that one receives and uses to launch oneself, to continue, and to endure; it is the same thrust that one passes on, and in doing so, one extends oneself in another form (i.e., through reproduction, or through less visible ways).

Long Life, Longevity

Chang Sheng (Ch'ang Shen)

長 生

Long Life means maintaining one's vitality in such a way that it is not used up. Nourished by the essential, having only natural life, thus reaching the full span of one's days and even going beyond apparent limits to eternal life.

Liver

肝

Gan
(Kan)

In the flesh 肉 of the body, the liver is the raised pestle 干 ready to attack and to grind, but also to sustain and to support. It is, as well, the defending and protective shield, thrust into the ground in front of oneself. He who knows best how to deliver blows also knows best how to receive them.

The liver must control its warrior-like power so that it will not be carried away by its own aggressiveness.

The liver, like springtime, or like the east where the sun rises, represents the thrust of life. Being the first to appear, it is also the first to fall or to suffer blows, because it is in an exposed position on the front line. That is why it must be anchored firmly in the Water, in the essences, and in the wise prudence of the kidneys, in order to keep the fullness and the quality of the blood that tempers the liver's ardor and permits the *Hun* to inspire reflection calmly.

The liver's power clears the passageways, and it gives the thrust to movements and circulations in such a way that it reaches to the extremities of the body, the exterior as well as the heights. This dynamism, founded upon the kidneys, is expressed in all the circulations where a boost or a starting up is needed, either to evacuate, or to absorb and assimilate, or to pass an obstruction. This goes for materialized elements, like blood, as well as for psychic elements, such as the emotions.

The liver has authority over the muscular strength, giving rise to movements. It frees the surplus of blood necessary for movements, and in so doing it gives dynamism, bringing suppleness, strength, and precision to the movements.

The fingernails and toenails extend to the exterior this alliance of strength and suppleness proper to Wood and to the liver. Also the eye, which projects far the flash of a glance and the grasp of a man, expresses the power of Wood's diffusion and extension. The eye is the orifice of the liver.

Many aspects of sexuality are in relationship with the liver: images, emotions, liberation of blood to fill erectile tissue, pulsation of life, and power of desire.

The liver is given the charge of being commander of armies. Analysis of circumstances and conception of plans proceed from there.

Suwen, Chapter 8

The liver is the rooting of one's capacity to stop at the outer limit; it is the dwelling-place of the *Hun*. Its flowering aspect is at the nails; the power of its fullness is in the muscular forces; it vivifies blood and breaths. . . . It is young *yang* within *yang*. It is in free communication with the breaths of springtime.

Suwen, Chapter 9

The eastern quadrant generates the wind. The wind generates wood. Wood generates acid. Acid generates the liver. The liver generates the musculature. The musculature generates the heart. The liver has mastery over the eye. . . . Among the colors it is blue-azure. Among the musical notes it is the note *jue*. Among the sounds it is the shout. Among the reactive movements to change it is contraction. . . .

Suwen, Chapter 5

Its domestic animal is the rooster; its grain is wheat . . . its odor is rancid.

Suwen, Chapter 4

When man is at rest, the blood returns to the liver. When the liver has received blood, one can see. . . .

Suwen, Chapter 10

Lung   Fei

肺

The lung is that which, in flesh 肉 , is analogous to branching plants 巿 that creep and divide without standing upright.

The lung, then, is abundance and prosperity, with a certain impulsiveness and rapidity in the vital force that is expressed by multiplying and reproducing. Order must be brought to this power of proliferation that extends everywhere and invades the territory all the way to the extremities.

The lung is the "master of breaths"; it directs and gives rhythm to respiration as well as to all circulations. This makes it assistant to the heart and master of the nose. It frees the breaths gathered in the middle of the chest, in order to disseminate them to the outer boundaries of the body: to the skin and body hair, the parts of the bodily structure that are animated by the same movement as the lung.

The skin, holding the body hair, sets the limit to the diffusion and expansion of the breaths and the corporeal form. The skin holds in the vitality while permitting productivity. The rhythms given by the lung animate the skin's respiration; the opening and closing of the well-managed pores prevent unwarranted loss of liquids, essences, and breaths to the outside.

To stop something and bring it back toward the inside is the appropriate movement of autumn, time of harvesting and gathering in. It is the movement of Metal, which condenses and compresses by pulling in and pushing down.

Placed at the top of the trunk, the lung surmounts like a canopy all the other organs. It exercises its downward pressure upon the humid vapors. Cooled and condensed into droplets by the lung's care, the liquids descend to the base of the trunk where they come under the control of the kidneys and the urinary bladder. The lung thus regulates the progress of liquids.

> The lung is given the charge of being minister and chancelor; the regulation of the pathways of animation proceeds from it.
>
> *Suwen*, Chapter 8

> The lung is the trunk where the breaths are rooted, the residence of the *Po*. Its flowering aspect is in the body hair; the power of its fullness is in the skin. It is great *yin* within *yang* (sub-diaphragmatic region). It is in free communication with the breaths of autumn.
>
> *Suwen*, Chapter 9

> The lung guarantees the free communication and regulation of the waterways.
>
> *Suwen*, Chapter 21

The western quadrant generates dryness. Dryness generates metal. Metal generates the acrid taste. The acrid taste generates the lung. The lung generates skin and body hair. Skin and body hair generate the kidneys. The lung has mastery over the nose. . . . Among the colors it is white; among the musical notes it is the note *shang*. Among the sounds it is weeping. Among the reactive movements to change it is coughing.

Suwen, Chapter 5

Its domestic animal is the horse. Its grain is rice. . . . Its odor is pungent.

Suwen, Chapter 4

Nature   Xing (Hsing)

性

The heart 心 and life 生 : one's proper nature, that which is natural.

Oppression and   Chou You
Sorrow   (Ch'ou Yu)

愁憂

Chou. When ears of corn 禾 have been ripened by the summer's fire 火 , it is autumn 秋 . But autumn as felt by the heart 心 can be a kind of tedious oppression and despondent melancholy where all is dreary, distressing, and hopeless. One is morose, for the heart is unable to take interest in anything. No longer is anything germinating or growing.

You. To drag everywhere 攵 a heart 心 and a head 頁 preyed upon by black worries is sorrow, burden, unhappiness, troubles, and world-weariness, where one plods beneath the weight of somber thoughts and heavy cares.

This suffering is a burden that adds heaviness to most of the other feelings, making their resolution or dissolution more difficult, thus leading to depression.

Po
(P'o) 魄

The *Po* are sensate souls, vegetative Spirits.

They are Spirits of Earth 鬼 which are animated by the same movement as is the color white *bai* 白 .

White can represent pure, total light or, as it does here, the spark of light from the setting sun, the gleam of cold metal, or the brightness of dried bones in the earth. In these latter examples, white is the color corresponding to autumn, to the west, the element Metal, and the lung. It is the opposite of the greenery appropriate to springtime, the east, the element Wood, and the liver.

Thus, as the opposite of essences *jing* 精 that rise and disperse lightly in the body, charged with the elements of vitality, the residues *Po* 粕 become concentrated, and they descend all the way to the complete evacuation of the elements that cannot be utilized for vital maintenance. This evacuation is made through the anus, also called "The Gate of the *Po*."

Their dwelling place in the body is the lung (see Lung).

(See also *Hun*).

Reflection   Lü

Project, conceptual plan, meditation; to reflect, to consider attentively, to conjecture, to estimate, to premeditate, to take to heart, to be careful; solicitude, preoccupation, doubt, uncertainty.

The character is a tiger's stripes 虍 enveloping thought 思.

The tiger leaps powerfully and far. He lands precisely, and he pins his prey to the ground. The same tiger remains immobile, even to his eyes, which watch without blinking for hours on end. He waits. His stripes signal his power. Concentrated repose and the unleashing of calculated movement are two aspects of the same virtue, always concentrated equally. These two aspects stand out in the regular pattern of alternating colors on fine, healthy fur.

The reunion of the two components (tiger's stripes and thought) gives to thought a watchful consideration, indeed even preoccupation, but one that permits the mind to take its risks, to calculate its estimations, and to plan with full awareness.

Reflection is often placed in relation to the liver and to the element Wood. The *Hun*, who are sheltered by the liver, give thought its powerful elevation and analytical correctness. The impetuous leap proper to the Wood sweeps away uncertainties, prevents stagnation of thought and the compulsion of repetition, and leads to the appropriate decision.

Si lü (szu lü) 思慮, to reflect intensely, to be preoccupied: worry and preoccupation.

Sadness and Grief

Bei Ai (Pei Ai)

悲·哀

Bei. The heart 心 rejects (itself) 非 . The person is back-to-back with himself in his heart, held prey by contradiction, denial, indeed by negativity. The exhaustion resulting from this sterile clash destroys the breaths in the region of the heart and lung. The struggle ruptures the communications emanating from the heart and cuts off the joy of life. The blockage leads to weakness, and distress becomes desolation.

Ai. Wails, groans, and lamentations coming from the mouth 口 of one who is dressed in the special garments 衣 of mourning. Grief experienced at the loss of a dear one; the sadness of mourning, shown publicly.

Sadness, corresponding to the lung, is perversion of the movement of Metal. The normal movement of Metal is condensation and concentration in order to bring the riches of life back into one's interior. In grief this movement becomes compression that crushes the heart, interfering with the circulation of a blood of diminishing quality, as well as with the expansion of the Spirits. This obstruction destroys both the liquids and the breaths of the lung. One dries up from grief, as one refuses to revive one's life, a revival incited by the liver (movement of Wood).

Spirits   Shen

神

Spirits. Divinities. The vital principle. Something marvelous.

The alternating expression of natural forces 申 (⽥) unfolds under the authority of influences from above 示 . Heaven thus penetrates and instructs all of humankind.

The Spirits are Heaven within us. They conduct us and guard us, and we must guard them.

(See also Essences/Spirits.)

There are also:

(Luminous radiance   Shen Ming
of the) Spirits

神 明

When the Spirits find natural Virtue, they make it shine. The conduct and meaning of life are illuminated by a resplendent flash of what is specifically celestial within us: the Spirits. The radiant activity of the Spirits is distributed by the auxiliaries subordinated to the power of the heart. The result is perceptible in all aspects of life, in virtuous and effective conduct, in bright and clear eyes, and in a fresh pink complexion. . . .

Spleen 脾

Pi (P'i)

In the flesh 肉 the spleen is analagous to an ordinary pot 卑 for daily use. A hard-working servant, the spleen toils unceasingly at tasks that have no glory, but that are enormously vital to the conduct of life.

The spleen corresponds to the central region, to the moment of passage from one season to another, at the center of permutations. Like the earth, it is the place where everything intersects, is accepted to be transformed, and goes off again in all directions in a new form. The earth receives all sorts of seeds and allows all the diverse plants and grains to grow, for the nourishment of living beings. The spleen receives alimentation and makes essential constituents assimilable by the organism, thanks to its work of transformation in digestion. The spleen then distributes these nutrients, these juices, these essences to all of the *zang*, and to each sector of the body. In this way vitality is constantly renewed.

As the center of equilibrium and like a turntable, the spleen maintains the balance of the exchanges, tensions and distributions. As place of passage, it is the liaison between the diverse components of an individual. Purveyor of new essences, it shapes the forms: the bodily form which is flesh; the mental form which is thought. It shapes the flesh and all parts of the organism through reconstruction and nutrition. It shapes the form of blood by the juices that are the basis of the blood. It shapes the form of the lips which surround the mouth (orifice of the spleen) and reflect the general condition of the flesh of the body. The mouth brings into the body the nourishment that comes from the earth.

As the earth, in order to be fertile, needs to be irrigated but not soaked, warmed but not burned, the spleen is penetrated with humidity that evaporates and rises continuously, so as not to encumber or hamper it. Between heart and kidneys, the spleen is the intersection of above and below, of Heaven and Earth. It is the fecund middle.

> The spleen and stomach are given the charge of being the barns and granaries. The five tastes come from there.
>
> *Suwen*, Chapter 8

The spleen, with the stomach, large intestine, small intestine, triple heater, and urinary bladder, is the rooting of the barns and granaries, the dwelling place of reconstruction. It is given the name "utensil." It is able to make the transformations that give residues and dregs, to convey the tastes, and to effect enterings and exitings. Its flowering aspect is at the four whites (corners) of the lips; the power of its fullness is in the flesh. It belongs to the supreme *yin*; it is in free communication with the breaths of the earth.

Suwen, Chapter 9

The central region generates humidity. Humidity generates earth. Earth generates the sweet taste. The sweet taste generates the spleen. The spleen generates the flesh. Flesh generates the lung. The spleen has mastery over the mouth . . . Among the colors it is earth-yellow. Among the musical notes it is the note *gong*. Among the sounds it is singing. Among the reactive movements to change it is belching.

Suwen, Chapter 5

Its domestic animal is the ox; its grain is millet . . . its odor is fragrant.

Suwen, Chapter 4

The spleen is the "Trunk of Posterior Heaven," and the "Gushing spring of transformations that produce blood and breaths."

Thought

Si

思、

(Szu)

Thought, conception, worries, concerns, obsession; to reflect, to consider, to remember.

The character shows the heart ᗯ below the cranial box 囟 that encloses the brain. The good relationship of the heart (and the Spirits dwelling there) with the brain allows thought to develop. Chapter 10 of *Lingshu* strongly indicates the direct liaison between the heart and the brain. This connection may pass through the tongue and the eye.

The heart permits internal fidelity, and the brain permits the good functioning of the orifices that communicate with the exterior. Brain marrow is constituted from the finest and subtlest essences, manifesting the original and hidden power of the kidneys in the radiant heights of the body.

Thought permits us to grasp and to link together in a firm line the elements of reason or of consideration. With acuity and penetration, thought goes to the deepest presented realities in a way that permits a knowing of the facts that leads to conjecture and planning.

Thought is related to the spleen and to the element Earth. Earth receives all of the sown seeds, in order to nourish them and ripen them, giving to each that which it needs. Earth permits the mixing and communicating of that which comes into its bosom; thus can water nourish vegetation and transform it into sap.

Thought, the spleen, and the Earth element permit circulations and permutations, free interpenetrations that allow the taking on of form.

Virtue   De
德   (Te)

Virtue is the uprightness 直 and the authenticity 真 of the heart 心 as it moves along 彳

Virtue *de* 德, is habitually placed in relationship with its homophone *de* 得 which means: to have received, to obtain, to possess, to attain in deep agreement.

Through virtue one both finds and possesses oneself.

Virtue gives authenticity to the actions of the one who possesses virtue. Knowledge without virtue is worthless. Virtue is good to everything and everyone and tirelessly provides appropriate results at every level.

If you are humanly virtuous, you will fulfill your responsibilities to everyone's satisfaction, and no one will find fault with your conduct.

If, initiated (into the mysteries), you evolve to the outer human limits, the Virtue of the Way will fill you to the bottom of your heart and will give you effectiveness and limitless perception.

Will
志

Zhi
(Chih)

Wish, design, goal, aspiration.

The intent in the heart 心 persists and develops, the way a plant begins to rise upward from the soil 士 (屮).

The movement of the heart is oriented continuously toward a goal; the plant represents the process of life's development. The heart takes on the power and tension of the phallus, as the plant represents the vigor of its stem.

The expression that unites will and intent brands fundamentally the orientation of all animation that begins in a well-constructed and inspired mental state.

There are multiple expressions joining not only intent to will, but also some of the other notions presented in *Lingshu*, Chapter 8. The variety of meanings permits us to grasp better the specificity of each character:

Zhi yi 志意 , will and intent: will, design (plan).

Yi zhi 意志 , intent and will: willingness, intention.

Zhi qi 志氣 , will and breaths: determination, the strength of soul in the character.

Yi qi 意氣 , intent and breaths: the state of the soul, morality, disposition, caprice, fantasy.

Xin zhi 心志 , heart and will: willpower, determination, resolution.

Xin yi 心意 , heart and intent: idea, thought, intention.

Shen zhi 神志 , Spirits and will: consciousness (awareness, knowledge).

Sheng yi 生意 , life and intent: vitality, commerce, human affairs.

Zang
(Tsang)

Organs/
Viscera

臟, 藏

Thesaurization, the active guarding of the Essences.

In a human, this guarding or storage is made in Five different and complementary ways, in the image of the Five Elements out of which Earth fashions all that exists. The Five *Zang* (liver, heart, spleen, lung, kidneys) are the Five command centers that order all of the vital movements, under the inspiration of the Spirits, and of the specific expressions of the spiritual power within each *zang*: the Spirits for the heart; the *Hun* for the liver; the *Po* for the lung; the Intent *yi* for the spleen; and the Will *zhi* for the kidneys. The *zang* capture the essences and work them in such a way that out of these transformations, the specific breaths are released that express the proper movement of each *zang*, each element, within the organism. The synergy of the *zang* is the center of the being and is manifested by the heart. The *zang* are solid and can be impregnated only by the essences, which are subtle, impalpable, and ready for all transformations. This is why the *zang* are also called the "full organs" or the "treasure organs."

General Index

The most commonly used Romanizations are given here for the Chinese characters: pinyin first; Wade-Giles in parentheses; followed by the principal page numbers in the text.

Index of
Proper Names
and
Names of Works

Art of War–Sunzi bingfa 孫子兵法 *(Sun Tzu Ping Fa)*, a treatise of military art, the classic of strategy, written around the fourth century B.C.

Book of Changes–Yijing 易經 *(I Ching)*, one of the Five Classics presenting, in sixty-four hexagrams, the vital fluctuations.

Book of History: The Annals –Shujing 書經 *(Shu Ching)*, one of the Five Classics, treating Chinese history from its origins to the middle of the Zhou dynasty.

Book of Music–Yueji 樂記 *(Yueh Chi)*, one of the treatises of the **Liji, Book of Rites.**

Book of Odes–Shijing 詩經 *(Shih Ching)*, one of the Five Classics, composed of poems.

Book of Rites–Liji 禮記 *(Li Chi)*, one of the Five Classics, dealing with order in human society.

Book of the Way and the Virtue, see *Laozi*.

Daodejing 道德經 *(Tao Te Ching)*, see *Laozi*.

Doctrine of the Mean–Zhongyong 中庸 *(Chung Yung)*, one of the Four Canonical Books of the Confucian School.

Guanzi 管子 *(Kuan Tzu)*, syncretic work composed between the fourth and first centuries B.C.

Huainanzi 淮南子 *(Huai Nan Tzu)*, syncretic work of the second century B.C.

Laozi 老子 *(Lao Tzu)*, legendary author of the *Daodejing, Book of the Way and the Virtue*, the most famous work of Daoism.

Lingshu 靈樞 *(Ling Shu)*, see *Neijing*.

Ma Shi 馬時 *(Ma Shih)*, one of the principal commentators of the *Neijing*.

Neijing 内經 *(Nei Ching)*, the basic work of Chinese Medicine, written between the fourth century B.C. and the ninth century A.D., and ordinarily composed of the *Suwen*, in the Wang Bing compilation (Tang), and of the *Lingshu* in the compilation of the Song era.

Qi Bo 歧伯 *(Ch'i Po)*, celestial Master, one of the great protagonists of the *Neijing*, the Yellow Emperor's interlocutor and professor.

Shang-yin 商殷 *(Shang Yin)*, name of the second Chinese dynasty; normally called Shang from its founding (1765 B.C.)

to the time of Emperor Pan Geng (1401 B.C.), and Yin from the time of the latter emperor until its fall (middle of the twelfth century B.C.).

Spring and Autumn Annals of Master Lü–Lüshi chunqiu 呂氏春秋 (**Lü Shih Ch'un Ch'iu**), the Springtimes and Autumns of Sir Lü, the sum of knowledge, written at the behest of Lü Buwei, around the middle of the third century B.C.

Suwen 素問 (**Su Wen**), see **Neijing**.

Taisu 太素 (**T'ai Su**), one of the great compilations of the canonical medical texts (**Sui Dynasty**), by Yang Shangshan.

Tao te king 道德經, see **Laozi**.

Wang Bing 王冰 (**Wang Ping**), one of the principal commentators of the **Suwen**, and also the editor of the present version.

Xunzi 荀子 (**Hsün Tzu**), Confucian philosopher (third century B.C.).

Yellow Emperor, Huangdi 黃帝 (**Huang Ti**), mythical emperor under whose patronage are placed, in the Han period, the sciences and arts of life (medicine, sexuality, etc.).

Zhang Jiebin 張介賓 (**Chang Chieh-Pin**), one of the principal commentators of the **Neijing**, author of a work rearranging this classic according to theme, the **Leijing** 類經 (**Lei Ching**).

Zhang Zhicong 張志聰 (**Chang Chih-Ts'ung**), one of the main commentators of the **Neijing**.

Zhuangzi 莊子 (**Chuang Tzu**), one of the very great Taoist philosophical authors (fourth century B.C.).

About the Authors and Translator

CLAUDE LARRE, S.J., studied Chinese in Beijing and Shanghai and lived in Japan and Vietnam for many years. He has a doctorate in Philosophy and Sinology from the University of Paris and degrees in Chinese, Japanese and Vietnamese Studies and Languages. He has written extensively on different aspects of Chinese culture, specializing in translating Daoist texts and Chinese medical texts. He is the founder of the Ricci Institute in Paris and director of the European School of Acupuncture.

ELISABETH ROCHAT DE LA VALLÉE is the senior lecturer of the European School of Acupuncture and a member of the Ricci Institute. She holds degrees in Philosophy and the Classics and in Chinese Studies. Madame Rochat de la Vallée has worked with Claude Larre for twenty years as a researcher and translator and has exceptional knowledge of the medical classics, grounded by her experience as an acupuncture practitioner.

Both Claude Larre and Elisabeth Rochat de la Vallée have published books and translations on Chinese philosophy and Chinese Traditional Medicine. They lecture in many countries in Europe, as well as in America.

SARAH STANG holds degrees from Sophie Newcomb College, La Sorbonne, and the Traditional Acupuncture Institute. She maintains an acupuncture practice in Washington, D.C. and is the translator and editor of books and articles, including *Survey of Traditional Chinese Medicine* (Larre, Schatz, and Rochat de la Vallée).

Other Works by the Authors of *Rooted in Spirit*

Published by the Traditional Acupuncture Foundation and the Ricci Institute:
Survey of Traditional Chinese Medicine; Symphony of the Yellow Emperor

Published by Monkey Press, England:
The Way of Heaven

Transcripts of seminars published by Monkey Press:
Secret Treatise of the Spiritual Orchid; The Lung; The Kidneys; Spleen/ Stomach; Heart Master, Triple Heater; The Heart; The Liver

The Ricci Institute

The Paris Ricci Institute was founded and directed by Father Claude Larre. For over twenty years its two main branches of activity have been sinological studies and social work. The sinological branch covers three areas: teaching, research, and publication.

The teaching of the Ricci Institute comprises regularly scheduled courses in Paris, as well as seminars in other French cities and in other countries (Germany, England, Belgium, Canada, The United States, Ireland, Israel, Italy, Sweden, Switzerland, and others). The courses are taught in French or English.

The Ricci Institute's research covers the study, translation, and presentation (with commentaries) of the Chinese classical texts, or the subjects of Taoism and Medicine, in particular. It also includes work on the *Grand Ricci,* an encyclopedic dictionary of the Chinese language. This latter work is done in collaboration with the Taipei Ricci Institute. This monumental work of more than 250,000 entries will appear in 1997/98 in both book form and CD-ROM.

The Ricci Institute publications deal with the mind and behavior of the Chinese as seen through their books and their life. They include *The Book of the Way and the Virtue* of Laozi, the most important parts of Zhuangzi and Huainanzi, and the essentials of the medical classics: the *Huangdi Neijing Suwen* and the *Lingshu.* In addition to co-publications with French, English, and Italian publishers, the Ricci Institute Installments (*Les Fascicules de l'Institut Ricci*), analyses of major philosophical and medical texts from the classical Chinese literature, a new series, *Les Varietes Sinologiques,* is published in both Paris and Taipei.

The three Ricci Institutes (Paris, San Francisco, and Taipei) founded the International Ricci Association (A.I.R.), which federates the Jesuit bodies that deal with Chinese life and culture.

The Ricci Institute and the European School of Acupuncture work together in teaching, research, and publication. Chinese thought is their observation tower. From there they observe human life as it unfolds against the background of the universe.

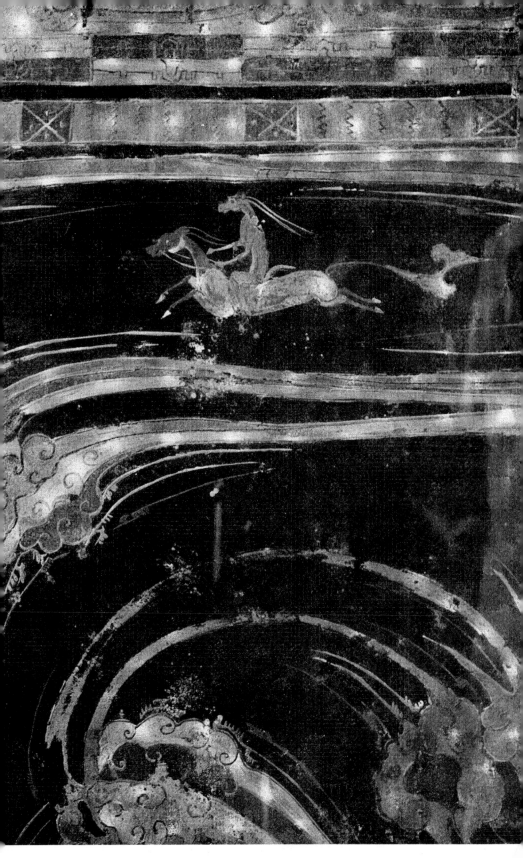

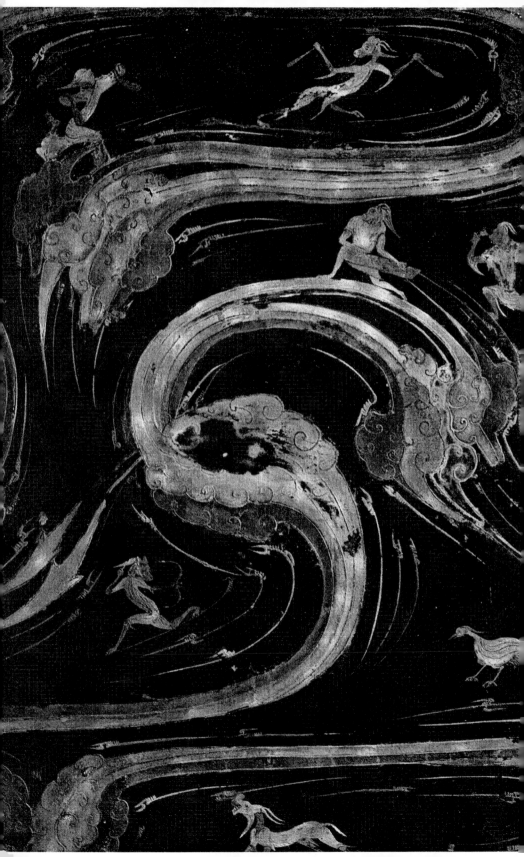